History of Toxicology and Environmental Health

History of Toxicology and Environmental Health

Toxicology in Antiquity, Volume II

Philip Wexler

AMSTERDAM • BOSTON • HEIDELBERG • LONDON
NEW YORK • OXFORD • PARIS • SAN DIEGO
SAN FRANCISCO • SINGAPORE • SYDNEY • TOKYO

Academic Press is an imprint of Elsevier

Academic Press is an imprint of Elsevier
32 Jamestown Road, London NW1 7BY, UK
525 B Street, Suite 1800, San Diego, CA 92101-4495, USA
225 Wyman Street, Waltham, MA 02451, USA
The Boulevard, Langford Lane, Kidlington, Oxford OX5 1GB, UK

Notices
Knowledge and best practice in this field are constantly changing. As new research and
experience broaden our understanding, changes in research methods, professional practices,
or medical treatment may become necessary.

Practitioners and researchers must always rely on their own experience and knowledge in
evaluating and using any information, methods, compounds, or experiments described herein.
In using such information or methods they should be mindful of their own safety and the safety
of others, including parties for whom they have a professional responsibility.

To the fullest extent of the law, neither the Publisher nor the authors, contributors, or editors,
assume any liability for any injury and/or damage to persons or property as a matter of products
liability, negligence or otherwise, or from any use or operation of any methods, products,
instructions, or ideas contained in the material herein.

British Library Cataloguing in Publication Data
A catalogue record for this book is available from the British Library

Library of Congress Cataloging-in-Publication Data
A catalog record for this book is available from the Library of Congress

ISBN: 978-0-12-801506-3

For Information on all Academic Press publications
visit our website at http://store.elsevier.com/

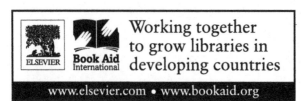

Working together
to grow libraries in
developing countries

www.elsevier.com • www.bookaid.org

TOXICOLOGY IN ANTIQUITY

Dedication—For Nancy, Yetty, Will, Jake, and Lola

With appreciation to the Toxicology History Association and the scholarly contributors to this series

Many thanks, as well, to Elsevier, in particular Molly McLaughlin, for expertly navigating us through the publication terrain.

CONTENTS

LIST OF CONTRIBUTORS

S. Waseemuddin Ahmed
Department of Pharmacognosy, Faculty of Pharmacy, University of Karachi, Karachi, Sindh, Pakistan

George Androutsos
History of Medicine Department, Medical School, National and Kapodistrian University of Athens, Athens, Greece

Iqbal Azhar
Department of Pharmacognosy, Faculty of Pharmacy, University of Karachi, Karachi, Sindh, Pakistan

Carl de Borhegyi
Independent researcher, USA
Previously associated with Liberal Arts department of Southwestern Michigan College, Dowagiac, MI, USA

Suzanne de Borhegyi-Forrest
Independent scholar, USA
Previously associated with Native American Arts, Brinton Museum of Western History, Big Horn, Wyoming; The Albuquerque Museum, Albuquerque, NM; The Wyoming Council on the Humanities, Laramie, Wyoming; The New Mexico Council on the Humanities, Albuquerque, New Mexico, USA

David Hillman
Classical Languages, St. Mary's University, USA

Evelyn Höbenreich
Institute of Roman Law and Antique History of Law, University of Graz, Graz, Austria

Mark A. Hoffman
Entheomedia.org, Taos, NM, USA

Yan Liu
History of Science, Harvard University, Cambridge, MA, USA

Zafar Alam Mahmood
Department of Pharmacognosy, Faculty of Pharmacy, University of Karachi, Karachi, Sindh, Pakistan

László Makra
Department of Climatology and Landscape Ecology, University of Szeged, Szeged, Hungary

Adrienne Mayor
Classics and History and Philosophy of Science and Technology, Stanford University, Stanford, CA, USA

Giunio Rizzelli
Roman Law, University of Foggia, Foggia, Italy

Carl A. P. Ruck
Classical Studies, Boston University, Boston, MA, USA

Michael Slouber
Liberal Studies, Western Washington University, Bellingham, WA, USA

Susan Stewart
Independent scholar, UK

Alain Touwaide
Institute for the Preservation of Medical Traditions and Smithsonian Institution, Washington, DC, USA

Gregory Tsoucalas
History of Medicine Department, Medical School, National and Kapodistrian University of Athens, Athens, Greece

Henry Ford was famously contemptuous of history. He is on record as saying, "History is more or less bunk. It's tradition. We don't want tradition. We want to live in the present and the only history that is worth a tinker's damn is the history we make today." Personally I prefer George Santayana's view: "...[W]hen experience is not retained, as among savages, infancy is perpetual. Those who cannot remember the past are condemned to repeat it." But how relevant is historical toxicology? What can we modern toxicologists (and our regulatory authorities) learn from the past? One important lesson is that toxicity can affect people anywhere, in any society, at any level, and for many years, without anyone being aware of it. Toxic effects on the brain may be responsible for misjudgments by political leaders that can have disastrous consequences. Toxicity may have caused the fall of empires. Jerome Nriagu [1] has argued in his 1983 book that "lead poisoning contributed to the decline of the Roman empire." Louise Cilliers, in Volume 1 of this series, though, disagrees with Nriagu's conclusion. Thus, we must consider further the Roman emperors' possible exposure to other toxicants described by Cilliers and Retief in an earlier article [2]. Maybe excessive wine consumption was enough to explain the emperors' self-destructive behavior. Maybe the effects of ethanol were supplemented by the effects of opium, widely used in ancient Rome as a soporific and an analgesic as well as an aid to digestion [2]. There is clearly still much scope for further research in this area.

Another empire that may have suffered the consequences of toxicity at the highest level is that of China. It seems possible that the latter days and decisions of the Chinese Emperor Qin Shi Huang may have been adversely affected by exposure to mercury. According to the historian Sima Qian, this emperor was buried in a mausoleum with 100 rivers of flowing mercury in addition to his now famous "terra cotta army." Reportedly, Qin Shi Huang died as a result of ingesting mercury pills, prescribed by his alchemists and court physicians in order to make him immortal [3]. It is not unreasonable to suppose, based on his interest in flowing mercury, which probably was to be found in his palace as well as his mausoleum, that some time before his death he was already suffering from mercury poisoning and that his mental function and judgment were impaired as a consequence. It is also likely that his son, the succeeding Emperor Qin Er Shi, had suffered exposure to mercury in his father's palace and that this led to his ill-judged decisions—for example, his command to lacquer the city walls [4]. In any event, his incompetence led to revolt, he was forced to commit suicide, and the Qin Dynasty and Empire came to an end, with the Qin capital being destroyed by rebels [4].

With these thoughts in mind, all toxicologists and all those concerned with human health, the environment, and the possible influence of toxic human environments on our political leaders must welcome the insights from history that this first volume and succeeding volumes in this new series of publications will bring. Frequently, I hear toxicologists remark that they might have reached better conclusions in the past "with the benefit of hindsight." Now that this series will give us the all the benefit of hindsight, no doubt "better conclusions" will follow.

John Duffus
The Edinburgh Centre for Toxicology

REFERENCES

[1] Nriagu JO. Saturnine gout among Roman aristocrats. Did lead poisoning contribute to the fall of the Empire? N Engl J Med 1983;308(11):660–3.

[2] Cilliers L, Retief FP. Poisons, poisoning and the drug trade in ancient Rome. Akroterion 2000;45:88–100.

[3] Wright DC. The history of China. Greenwood Publishing Group, Westport, CT; 2001; 264 pp. ISBN 0-313-30940-X.

[4] Hardy G, Kinney AB. The establishment of the Han Empire and Imperial China. Greenwood Publishing Group, Westport, CT; 2005; 170 pp. ISBN 031332588X.

In the realm of communicating any science, history, though critical to its progress, is typically a neglected backwater. This is unfortunate, as it can easily be the most fascinating, revealing, and accessible aspect of a subject which might otherwise hold appeal for only a highly specialized technical audience. Toxicology, the science concerned with the potentially hazardous effects of chemical, biological, and certain physical agents, has yet to be the subject of a full-scale historical treatment. Overlapping with many other sciences, it both draws from and contributes to them. Chemistry, biology, and pharmacology all intersect with toxicology. While there have been chapters devoted to history in toxicology textbooks, and journal articles have filled in bits and pieces of the historical record, this new monographic series aims to further remedy the gap by offering an extensive and systematic look at the subject from antiquity to the present.

Since ancient times, men and women have sought security of all kinds. This includes identifying and making use of beneficial substances while avoiding the harmful ones, or mitigating harm already caused. Thus, food and other natural products, independently or in combination, which promoted well-being or were found to have drug-like properties and effected cures, were readily consumed, applied, or otherwise self-administered or made available to friends and family. On the other hand, agents found to cause injury or damage—what we might call *poisons* today—were personally avoided although sometimes employed to wreak havoc upon one's enemies.

While natural substances are still of toxicological concern, synthetic and industrial chemicals now predominate as the emphasis of research. Through the years, the instinctive human need to seek safety and avoid hazard has served as an unchanging foundation for toxicology, and will be explored from many angles in this series. Although largely examining the scientific underpinnings of the field, chapters will also delve into the fascinating history of toxicology and poisons in mythology, arts, society, and culture more broadly. It is a subject that has captured our collective consciousness.

The series is intentionally broad, thus the title *History of Toxicology and Environmental Health*. Clinical and research toxicology, environmental and occupational health, risk assessment, and epidemiology, to name but a few examples, are all fair game subjects for inclusion. Volumes 1 and 2 focus on toxicology in antiquity, taken roughly to be the period up to the fall of the Roman empire and stopping short of the Middle Ages, with which period future volumes will continue. These opening volumes will explore toxicology from the perspective of some of the great civilizations of the past, including Egypt, Greece, Rome, Mesoamerica, and China. Particular substances, such as harmful botanicals, lead, cosmetics, kohl, and hallucinogens, serve as the focus of other chapters. The role of certain individuals as either victims or practitioners of toxicity (e.g., Cleopatra, Mithridates, Alexander the Great, Socrates, and Shen Nung) serves as another thrust of these volumes.

History proves that no science is static. As Nikola Tesla said, "The history of science shows that theories are perishable. With every new truth that is revealed we get a better understanding of Nature and our conceptions and views are modified."

Great research derives from great researchers who do not, and cannot, operate in a vacuum, but rely on the findings of their scientific forebears. To quote Sir Isaac Newton, "If I have seen further it is by standing on the shoulders of giants."

Welcome to this toxicological journey through time. You will surely see further and deeper and more insightfully by wafting through the waters of toxicology's history.

Phil Wexler

CHAPTER 1

Murder, Execution, and Suicide in Ancient Greece and Rome

Alain Touwaide

The political, scientific, cultural, and artistic life of the ancient world may be highlighted by such remarkable individuals as Pericles (ca. 495–429 BCE), Aristotle (384–322 BCE), Thucydides (460–395 BCE), and Phidias (490–430 BCE) in Greece, and Augustus (63 BCE; *reign.* 27 BCE–15 CE), Pliny (23/4–79 CE), and Cicero (106–43 BCE), as well as by Pompeii's many fresco painters in the Roman world. It also seems to have been punctuated by treacherous murders, summary executions, and self-inflicted death for many reasons ranging from lovesickness to desperation and shame. Many illustrious individuals have been reported to have committed suicide: for example, the Athenian orator Demosthenes (384–322 BCE); the Egyptian Queen Cleopatra (69–30 BCE); even the philosopher Aristotle according to the ancient historian and philosopher Diogenes Laertius and the Byzantine lexicographer and historian of literature Hesychius; and the Carthaginian general Hannibal (247/6–183 BCE).

The case of the Athenian politician and general, Themistocles, (ca. 525–ca. 459) is revealing. According to historical accounts, he committed suicide by drinking bull's blood, which in antiquity was believed to be highly toxic (and it probably was due to toxins such as botulinum, anthrax, or others resident in cattle). As the story goes, after he defeated the Persian fleet attacking Athens in the Bay of Salamis in 480 BCE, Themistocles was banished from Athens for political reasons and escaped to Persia. There, King Artaxerxes I (*reign.* 465–424/3 BCE) ordered him to lead a military operation against Greece. Themistocles refused and reportedly committed suicide rather than betray his country. Closer examination of the story reveals, however, that following Themistocles's death (which probably was due to natural causes) its details were deliberately misinterpreted to save the reputation of an esteemed, victorious general

History of Toxicology and Environmental Health. DOI: http://dx.doi.org/10.1016/B978-0-12-801506-3.00001-7

turned traitor. To preserve the memory of his sacrifice, a statue was erected depicting Themistocles slaughtering a bull for sacrifice, thereby perpetuating the legend that he committed suicide rather than attack his native land.

Although suicide, murder, and execution were certainly a reality in ancient life, they were not necessarily as frequent occurrences as popular legend, political propaganda, or other ill-intentioned maneuvers would have us believe. At any rate, the use of lethal substances may be questioned. Often documentary evidence is anecdotal and cannot be corroborated for lack of supplementary and independent sources, or for presenting contradictory or implausible scenarios, as Cleopatra's death suggests. A suicide carried out through a cobra's organized biting seems to be more speculative than likely. Ancient medical literature credited cobra's venom with causing instant paralysis, leading to immediate death. A suicide with no suffering was ideal and would have certainly been the supposedly self-indulgent Cleopatra's choice. Nevertheless, it is highly improbable that a cobra could have been brought into her apartments without having been noticed. Cleopatra and Egypt were very important to the Roman Empire because of Egypt's rich resources, especially its abundant agricultural production, which Rome needed to feed its people. Indeed, Cleopatra herself was viewed as a precious political commodity. At the same time, because of her liaison with Marc Antony, who had been defeated by Octavius, the future Emperor Augustus, Cleopatra became politically undesirable. Under these conditions, Cleopatra was kept under strict control in her palace where she could easily be assassinated. Her assassination was extremely risky, for it could well have provoked mob action and have led to Rome's loss of control over Egypt. Crediting her with suicide—for reasons of desperation, political calculation, or any other reason—was the ideal coverup and so we will probably never know exactly how she died.

Murder was more often committed by stabbing than by poisoning. Caesar (100–44 BCE) is the best example. He was stabbed in plain light, in the Curia, by a group of conspirators, including his adoptive son ("Tu quoque, Brute, fili mi"—"You too, Brutus"). In many other cases, however, toxic substances were used. In the ancient Greek world, sovereigns who succeeded Alexander the Great and divided his empire showed a particular interest in poisoning. Antigonus Gonatas (ca. 320–239 BCE), king of Macedonia, Antiochus III (ca. 242–187 BCE), king of Seleucia, and Ptolemaeus IV Philopator, king of Egypt (ca. 244–205 BCE) were among such kings, together with Attalus III Philometer Evergetes, king of Pergamum (*reign*. 138–133 BCE). to whom Nicander dedicated one of his poems. According to historical sources, Attalus cultivated medicinal and toxic plants, including henbane, helle-bore, hemlock, and aconite. He is credited with testing their toxic proper-ties on individuals who had been sentenced to death. The purpose was not only to prepare poisons and to identify their lethal doses, but also–if not primarily–to make use of them, particularly in a time when political rivalry was intense and coups d'etat were not rare. The most famous among these Hellenistic kings who were manipulators of poisons is without doubt Mithradates VI Eupator, king of Pontus (133; *reign.* 120–63 BCE). An ambitious and unscrupulous politician, Mithradates had assassinated several members of his court and even members of his family (including his own mother) to preserve his throne. Furthermore, he fiercely opposed the Roman conquest of Asia Minor and inflicted severe defeat on Roman troops. Correctly fearing that he might be poiso-ned–whether by his own entourage or by the Romans–he absorbed increasing doses of all possible poisons to acquire immunity. He was so successful that, when he was eventually captured by the Romans in 63 BCE and he wanted to kill himself in order to escape the clutches of his captors, he consumed a poison that he always carried with him but did not die. He had no other recourse than to ask his slaves to run him through with a sword.

Poisons were no less common in Rome. As early as 449 BCE, the *Lex duodecim tabellarum* (Law of the Twelve Tables) prohibited poi-sons, thus clearly implying that they had been in use. The law probably did not have much effect, as a new one needed to be promulgated in 81 BCE: the famous *Lex Cornelia de sicariis et veneficis* (Cornelia Law on Assassins and Poisoners). Again, this new legislation did not neces-sarily prevent poisoning. Indeed, half a century later, the Latin poet Tibullus (ca. 55–19 BCE) wrote an elegy in which he recalled a sickness during which he thought he would die. Imploring mercy from Persephone, the Queen of the Underworld, he proclaimed that he did not poison anybody. Murder by poison even took place within the imperial palace, as is shown by the case of Claudius (10; emp. 41, d. 54 CE). Claudius was known to be fond of mushrooms, and so it was that he was served with an abundant plate of mushrooms, supposedly of boletus, but they might have been mixed with a poison. Whatever the toxic agent used, Claudius did die. It was his second wife, Agrippina (15–59 CE), who initiated plans to get Claudius out of the way so that her son Nero (37; emp. 54; d. 68) would become emperor. Claudius's poisoning was orchestrated by Agrippina in collusion with a woman named Locusta, who was supposedly from Gaul, had mastered the art of poisons, and had been sentenced to jail for poisoning. Taken out of prison, she helped engineer Claudius's murder. Ironically enough, she also prepared the poison that Nero himself would later use to kill himself. As for Locusta herself, she was executed under Emperor Galba (24; emp. 68–69), who, in turn, was killed by mutinous soldiers.

With rare exception, the exact nature of the poisons used for murder—whether they were prepared by an expert such as Locusta or by less competent assassins—is not known. The art of compounding poisons seems to have flourished during the first century BCE. Interestingly enough, this period also saw an unprecedented development of compound medicines. The origin of this therapeutic strategy is often attributed to Mithradates. However, a compound medicine appeared earlier in Nicander's *Theriaca*, which suggests that such a practice must have predated Mithradates. Whatever the case, the formula for the medicine mentioned in Nicander's *Theriaca* was refined by the Cretan Andromachus, who was Nero's personal physician. It thus seems that, during the first century CE and particularly during Nero's reign (54–68 CE), a substantial amount of research was done on compounding—and also administering—medicines and possibly poisons by mixing several substances, medicinal or toxic, respectively, together.

If the nature of poisons is unknown in many cases, it might be because poison had a special off-limits status in the ancient world, apart from the evident secrecy of criminal poisoning. Its manipulation was often attributed to individuals who were on the margins of society. Locusta is exemplary from that viewpoint. Women had no rights under Roman law but acquired status only by being married; Locusta was of foreign origin and consequently had even fewer legal rights than most Roman women. At any rate, she lost any possibility of acquiring an official status once she was condemned for her poisonings. Locusta's case was not unusual. Long before she appeared on the scene, the archetype of the individual at the margins of society who was a user of poisons had arrived in the person of the legendary Medea. A granddaughter of the sun god Helios and of the magician Circe, Medea was the daughter of the king of Colchis, living on the Black Sea, at the eastern edge of the Greek world, at the border of Scythia. She used her singular talents to manipulate poisons in various ways. She first laid eyes on Jason when he arrived at Colchis from Greece during his expedition to conquer the Golden Fleece; Medea instantly fell in love with him. But being the daughter of the local king, she could not even think of approaching this foreigner, and so she tried to commit suicide. She got hold of a poison defined only by its black color (actually the color of the death it was supposed to provoke), which, however, she did not drink because she was too frightened to do so. An additional deterrent to her taking the poison was her sister's admonition that by killing herself she would destroy a promising life. After Jason acquired the Golden Fleece and returned victorious to Medea's father, the two married and they had several children. Later, Jason fell in love with another woman. Plotting her revenge, Medea poisoned a tunic by dyeing it with a substance described with many details in literature, but more fictional than realistic. She offered this tunic to her rival who upon slipping it on died in severe pain. As further, complete revenge against Jason, immediately afterward Medea killed their children. Medea's legend was more paradigmatic than historical and was told to future generations to provide ethical guidelines. Indeed, the story aimed to show that poisoning out of jealousy was the typical act of irrational people, as Medea's murder of her own children demonstrated, whereas committing suicide out of lovesickness was more understandable. All the same, it was to be avoided since, for the youthful lover, it meant the end of a life that had just begun. In this view, the exact nature of the poison did not matter; poisoning was a concept rather than a particular tool.

Toxic substances had a special status in historical sources at the edge of reality and imagination. According to Theophrastus (372/0– ca. 288/6 BCE), a pupil of Aristotle and the compiler of the first work on botany (*Historia plantarum—Inquiries into plants*), skilled poisoners were able to prepare aconite in such a way that it would kill in a fixed time: two months, three months, and even one or two years—but this is likely a fiction. Nonetheless, in this same work, Theophrastus displays a genuine grasp of pharmacology in his description of how a contemporary of Aristotle, Thrasyas of Mantinea, mixed hemlock and poppy, thereby producing a poison that would kill without pain.

Although cases of poisoning have been attested to in written documents, their frequency should not be overstated. The same can probably also be said about execution. The execution of Socrates with hemlock in 399 BCE should not lead to the conclusion that poisons were common instruments of execution. Indeed, techniques other than poisoning were used. Seneca (ca. 1 CE−64 CE), who had been Nero's tutor, was condemned to death (actually, he was forced to commit suicide) for his supposed participation in a conspiracy against the emperor. Rather than take poison, Seneca chose to open his veins. Nevertheless, hemlock was said to be available in Masalia (present-day Marseilles) in a safe box for those who were condemned, as well as for others who chose to end their lives.

Information is no more specific for suicide than it is for murder. Again, we can look to mythology for precedents. One myth tells the story of Antheia, the wife of Proetus, the king of Tyrins, in continental Greece. The two had been married for many years and had several children. However, one day when the beautiful Bellerophon paid them a visit, Antheia fell in love with him. When Bellerophon spurned her advances, Antheia got her revenge by accusing him of attempting to rape her. Proetus thereupon expelled Bellerophon, who later returned to Tyrins after he was proven innocent of Antheia's charge. Upon his arrival, Antheia committed suicide through a means that is not specified in the literature. Contrary to Medea's account, suicide committed out of lovesickness was accepted: Antheia was not in her prime and so was unlike those whose young life would have ended before really getting started.

In historical times, many individuals, famous or not, committed suicide by poison. One of these individuals was the Carthaginian general, Hannibal. A fierce enemy of the Romans, Hannibal was defeated by them in 202 BCE. About to be captured by the Romans in 195, he fled to Asia Minor and was granted refuge first by the court of the poisoner king of Seleucia, Antiochus III, and subsequently by the king of Bithynia, Prusias I (ca. 230−182 BCE). When the Romans asked Prusias to extradite Hannibal, the general took poison from a ring he was wearing; the nature of this poison is not known, being referred to in ancient literature only by the imprecise term *venenum*.

There is an abundant body of ancient literature on poisons, starting with Nicander in Asia Minor, possibly in the second century BCE, proceeding to Galen (129–after [?] 216 CE) in Rome, and later to Oribasius (fourth century), Aetius (sixth century) in Byzantium, and Paul of Egina (seventh century) in Alexandria. Their works reflect a precise knowledge of poisons and their actions. These works are fundamentally medical in nature and devoted to the treatment of poisoning-, whether criminal or accidental, rather than being guides to the art of poisoning, although this knowledge of poisons could very well have been used by nonspecialists with criminal intentions. It is much more likely that knowledge of toxic substances to be used for suicide, assassination, and execution—apart from some notorious exceptions such as Socrates' death and Plato's description of it—circulated solely among a select group of professionals who sold their secrets, were hired as professional killers, or were state executioners. At the same time, common people likely possessed a rudimentary knowledge of poisons and their deadly use; women were even more likely to have such knowledge, as the use of abortifacients suggests. Such knowledge probably never made its way into learned medical literature, particularly because the authors of this literature were physicians who having sworn the Hippocratic oath pledged that they would not administer poisons.

SUGGESTED READINGS

Amberger-Lahrmann M, Schmöhl D, editors. Gifte. Geschichte der toxikologie. Berlin: Springer; 1988.

Arihan O, Karaoz Arihan S, Touwaide A. The case against Socrates and his execution. In: Wexler P, editor. History of toxicology and environmental health, toxicology in antiquity, vol. 1. Amsterdam: Elsevier; 2014. p. 69–82.

Cilliers L, Retief F. Poisons, poisoners, and poisoning in ancient Rome. In: Wexler P, editor. History of toxicology and environmental health, toxicology in antiquity, vol. 1. Amsterdam: Elsevier; 2014. p. 127–37.

de Maleissye J. Histoire du poison. Paris: François Bourin; 1991.

Golden CL The role of poison in Roman society. (PhD thesis), Chapel Hill, University of North Carolina; 2005.

Lewin L. Die Gifte in der Weltgeschichte. Toxikologisch, allgemeinverständliche untersuchungen der historischen quellen. Berlin: Julius Springer; 1920.

Martinetz D, Lohs K. Poison. Sorcery and science. Friend and Foe. Leipzig: Edition Leipzig; 1987.

Mayor A. Mithridates of Pontus and his universal antidote. In: Wexler P, editor. History of toxicology and environmental health, toxicology in antiquity, vol. 1. Amsterdam: Elsevier; 2014. p. 21–33.

Mayor A. Alexander the Great: A questionable death. In: Wexler P, editor. History of toxicology and environmental health, toxicology in antiquity, vol. 1. Amsterdam: Elsevier; 2014. p. 52–9.

Pichon-Vendueil E. Etude sur les pharmaques et venins de l'antiquité. Poisons de guerre, de chasse, de justice et de suicide des anciens peuples de l'Europe (Scythes, Hellènes, Italiotes, Celtes, Germains et Ibères). (PhD thesis), University of Bordeaux, Bordeaux; 1914.

Tsoucalas G, Sgantzos M. The death of Cleopatra: Suicide by snakebite or poisoned by her enemies? In: Wexler P, editor. History of toxicology and environmental health, toxicology in antiquity, vol. 1. Amsterdam: Elsevier; 2014. p. 11–20.

Touwaide A. Harmful botanicals. In: Wexler P, editor. History of toxicology and environmental health, toxicology in antiquity, Vol. 1. Amsterdam: Elsevier; 2014. p. 60–8.

Vuillet-A-Cilles C. Les empoisonnements dans l'antiquité chez les peuples indo-européens. (PhD thesis) University of Besançon, Besançon; 1986.

CHAPTER 2

Chemical and Biological Warfare in Antiquity

Adrienne Mayor

Biological weapons employ viable, living organisms, such as pathogens, venoms, and toxic plants, insects, or animals, while poisonous gases, dust, or smoke, and incendiary materials to burn, blind, choke, or asphyxiate foes constitute chemical weapons. In antiquity, a wide range of substances, from toxic plants and venomous insects and reptiles to infectious agents and noxious chemicals, were weaponized in Europe, the Mediterranean, North Africa, the Middle East, Central Asia, India, China, and the Americas. Natural toxins were exploited to wage the earliest forms of biological and chemical warfare. Literary and archaeological evidence for the concept and practice of toxic warfare can be traced back to thousands of years. For example, in Asia Minor cuneiform tablets of about 1200 BC record that the Hittites deliberately drove victims of plague into enemy territory. True scientific understanding of toxicology, epidemiology, and chemistry were not required to carry out such practices, nor did the perpetrators need to possess advanced technology. Instead, the use of toxic arms and tactics was based on centuries of observation and experimentation with easily available toxic materials. A strategy based on attacking an opponent's biological vulnerabilities with poison could give a commander an advantage when his men faced troops that were superior in numbers, courage, military prowess, or technology. Nevertheless, the use of toxic weapons entailed practical and ethical dilemmas even in antiquity.

The concept of poisoned projectiles is embedded in the ancient Greek language. *Toxicon*, the word for "poison," derives from *toxon*, the word for "arrow." It is likely that the first projectiles treated with poisonous substances were devised for hunting animals and later turned toward warfare. The bow and arrow was a highly effective delivery system for toxins at an early date. Even a scratch from a poisoned arrowhead or spear could be fatal.

History of Toxicology and Environmental Health. DOI: http://dx.doi.org/10.1016/B978-0-12-801506-3.00002-9

2.1 THE CONCEPT OF TOXIC WEAPONRY IN GRECO-ROMAN AND INDIAN MYTHOLOGY

Greek mythology offers further evidence of the antiquity of the concept of toxic weapons. The great mythic hero Hercules, for example, created the first biological weapon in Western literature. After destroying a terrible many-headed serpent, the Hydra, Hercules dipped his arrows in the monster's venom; thereafter his quiver was filled with a never-ending supply of Hydra-envenomed arrows. Homer's *Iliad*, an oral epic first written down in the eighth century BC, contains indirect allusions to the use of toxic projectiles in the legendary Trojan War. Homer described black (rather than red) blood oozing from wounds, doctors sucking out poisons from arrow wounds on the battlefield, and never-healing wounds: these details are hallmarks of poisoning by snake venom. In the *Odyssey* (2.225–30) Homer describes the Greek hero Odysseus seeking lethal plant juices to treat arrows intended for his enemies. According to ancient legend, Odysseus himself was killed by a poisoned weapon—a spear tipped with the toxic spine of the marbled stingray, a common species in the Mediterranean [1].

In the *Aeneid* (9.770–74), an epic poem by Virgil recounting the legendary history of Rome, poisoned spears were employed by the early Romans. Poisoned weapons also appear in the great mythological epic of India, the *Rig Veda*. These Greek and Indian myths and legends are thought to reflect the early invention of biological weaponry in ancient cultures. The mythic examples also offered models for and may have reflected the actual practice of chemical and biological warfare [1].

2.2 POISONS FROM PLANTS IN HISTORICAL WARFARE

In antiquity, dozens of toxic Eurasian plant species were known and used as medicines in very tiny dosages. These powerful plants were also gathered to make arrow poisons or other biological weaponry used in historical battles. Hellebore was one of the most popular plant drugs, classified by the ancient Greeks as black hellebore (the Christmas rose of the buttercup Ranunculaceae family, *Helleborus niger*) and white hellebore (the lily family, *Liliaceae*). Each of these two unrelated plants are laden with powerful chemicals that cause severe vomiting and diarrhea, muscle cramps, delirium, convulsions, asphyxia, and heart attack. Hellebore was the poison sought by

Odysseus in Homer's *Odyssey*, and it was one of the arrow drugs used by the Gauls, among other groups. Hellebore was also used to poison the wells of besieged cities (see Section 2.5).

Aconite or monkshood (wolfsbane) was another favorite plant toxin. Aconitum (buttercup family) contains the alkaloid aconitine, a dangerous poison. In high doses, it causes vomiting and paralyzes the nervous system, resulting in death. Aconite was employed by archers of both ancient Greece and India, and its use in warfare continued into modernity. In 1483, for example, in the war between the Spanish and the Moors, the Arab archers wrapped their arrow points with aconite-soaked cotton. During World War II, Nazi scientists experimented with aconitine-treated bullets [1].

Another arrow poison in antiquity was henbane (*Hyoscyamine niger*), a sticky, nasty-smelling weed containing the powerful narcotics hyoscyamine and scopolamine. Henbane causes violent seizures, psychosis, and death. Other plant juices used on projectiles in antiquity included yew (*Taxus*), hemlock (*Conium maculatum*), rhododendron, azalea, and deadly nightshade or belladonna, which causes vertigo, extreme agitation, coma, and death. According to Pliny the Elder, a natural historian of Rome in the first century AD, the archaic Latin word for deadly nightshade was *dorycnion*, "spear drug." Pliny (*Natural History* 21.177−79) noted that this fact indicated that the plant was used to treat weapons at a very early date in Italy.

2.3 SNAKE VENOM ARROWS

Snake venom was another dreaded arrow poison used by several groups in antiquity. Because snake venom is digestible it could be safely used for hunting game. But if venom could be introduced into the bloodstream of a human enemy, it would guarantee a painful death or a never-healing wound. Numerous poisonous snakes exist around the Mediterranean and in Africa and Asia. According to ancient Greek and Roman sources, archers who steeped their arrows in viper or snake venom included the Gauls, Dalmatians, and Dacians of the Balkans; the Sarmatians of Persia (Iran); the Getae of Thrace; the Slavs, Armenians, and Parthians, who lived between the Indus and Euphrates rivers; Indians; North Africans; and the Scythian nomads of the Black Sea region and the Central Asian steppes. According to

Strabo, a Greek geographer, the people of Ethiopia dipped their arrows "in the gall of serpents." Strabo also claimed that the arrow poison concocted by the Soanes of the Caucasus was so noxious that the odor alone was injurious. The Roman historian Silius Italicus (*Punica* 1.320–415) described envenomed arrows used by the archers of Morocco, Libya, Egypt, and Sudan. Ancient Chinese texts tell us that arrow poisons were also in use in China, and in the New World Native Americans used snake, frog, and plant poisons on projectiles for both hunting and warfare [1–3].

Simple and complex ways of making envenomed arrows are recorded in Greek and Latin texts. Snake venom crystallizes and so can cling and remain viable on wooden, bone, and metal points for a considerable time. One of the most feared arrow drugs in antiquity was the complicated *scythicon* created by the Scythians. They mixed venom with bacteriological pathogens from animal dung, human blood, and putrefying viper carcasses (Aelian, *On Animals* 9.15; Ovid, *Tristia; Letter from Pontus*). In even a superficial wound from a *scythicon*-treated arrow, the toxins would begin taking effect within an hour. Envenomation would be compounded by shock, and necrosis and suppuration would be followed by gangrene and tetanus. *Scythicon* ensured an agonizing death.

Several snake species were available to the Scythians: the steppe viper *Vipera ursinii renardi*, the Caucasus viper *Vipera kasnakovi*, the European adder *Vipera berus*, and the long-nosed or sand viper *Vipera ammodytes transcaucasiana*. The natural historian Aelian (third-century AD Rome) described one of the most fearsome poisons of India, derived from the venom and rotting carcasses of the so-called white-headed Purple Snake. From Aelian's detailed description, herpetologists identify the Purple Snake as the rare, white-headed viper discovered in South Asia in the late 1880s, *Azemiops feae*.

The army of Alexander the Great in his conquest of India in 327–325 BC encountered a different snake-venom weapon. According to the historians of his campaigns, Quintus Curtius, Diodorus of Sicily, and others, the defenders of Harmatelia (Mansura in today's Pakistan) had dipped their arrows and swords in an unknown snake poison. Any man who suffered even a slight wound felt immediately numb and experienced stabbing pains and convulsions. The victim's skin became pale and cold and he vomited bile. Soon, a black froth exuded from the wound. Purplish-green gangrene spread rapidly, followed by death. Modern historians have assumed that cobra venom was used at Harmatelia, but the very detailed descriptions of the ghastly symptoms and deaths suffered by Alexander's soldiers points to another snake. Cobra venom would bring a relatively painless death, from respiratory paralysis. But the common Russell's viper of Pakistan and India causes the very same symptoms suffered by Alexander's men: numbness, vomiting, severe pain, black blood, gangrene, and death [1].

2.4 PLAGUE AND CONTAGION

Modern historians have considered the Mongols' ploy of catapulting of bubonic plague victims over the walls at Kaffa on the Black Sea in AD 1346 as the first recorded act of biological warfare. But empirical understandings of contagion developed much earlier in history. The Hittites' use of plague was mentioned above. In another early example, in Mesopotamia in about 1770 BC cuneiform tablets warned that disease could be spread by fomites, infectious pathogens on clothing, bedding, and other items. Jewish legends about King Solomon suggested that he hid plague in sealed jars in the Temple of Jerusalem to infect Babylonian and Roman invaders. During the Peloponnesian War (fourth century BC), the Athenians suspected that the Spartans had spread the great plague (apparently smallpox) by poisoning their wells. The accusation shows that people feared such tactics, whether they really occurred or not.

The Latin phrase *pestilentia manu facta* ("manmade pestilence") was coined by Seneca (*On Anger* 2.9.3). Two incidents of deliberately transmitted contagion were reported during the reigns of Domitian (AD 90) and Commodus (AD 189). According to Dio Cassius (*Epitome* 67.11 and 73.14), saboteurs pricked people with tiny needles dipped in deadly substances, causing epidemics and panic. Whether true or not, such rumors play a role in bioterrorism. The Great Plague of AD 165–180 (again, probably smallpox), was spread from Babylon (modern Iraq) to Syria, Italy, and as far as Germany by Roman soldiers returning from the war undertaken to control Mesopotamia. According to historians of that era, the epidemic began when some Roman soldiers looted a treasure chest in an enemy temple in Babylonia. These historical accounts imply that the chest had been deliberately booby-trapped with plague-laden items, a plausible notion. The local population would have had some immunity to the epidemic while the invading Roman army would have been immunulogically naive and vulnerable. At the very least, the ancient reports demonstrate that the idea of deliberately spreading epidemics among the enemy was widely contemplated by that time [1].

In ancient India, Kautilya's *Arthashastra*, a warfare manual dating to the fourth century BC, suggested ways of infecting enemies with illnesses such as fevers, wasting lung disease, and rabies. The *Arthashastra* also gives numerous recipes for poisoning the food and water of the enemy [4].

2.5 POISONING WATER SOURCES AND FOOD SUPPLIES

Tainting water and food supplies was another ancient poison tactic. A legendary Greek account set in about 1000 BC tells how King Cnopus conquered Erythrae (western Turkey) by consulting a "witch" from Thessaly, Greece. Her strategy was to poison a sacrificial bull. She then tricked the Erythraeans into eating the poisoned meat. The enemy was easily routed by King Cnopus's army.

The earliest historically documented case of poisoning drinking water in Greece occurred in about 590 BC during the First Sacred War. Athens and allied city-states were besieging Kirrha, the strongly fortified town that controlled the road to Delphi, the site of the sacred Oracle of Apollo. Athens and her allies argued that Kirrha had offended the god and was therefore to be totally destroyed. To break the siege deadlock, the commander of the league of allies ordered his men to gather and crush a great quantity of hellebore plants, which grew in profusion in the area. They placed the hellebore in the water pipes supplying Kirrha. The soldiers manning the walls—and the entire population of Kirrha—fell violently ill after drinking the poisoned water. Athens and the league overran the city and slaughtered the combatants and the civilians alike. After the Sacred War, Athens and her allies had second thoughts. They agreed among themselves not to interfere with water supplies should they ever find themselves at war with each other [1].

At least one Roman general was known to have poisoned wells. Manius Aquillius ended a long-drawn-out war to quell insurrections in the Roman province of Asia Minor in 129 BC by pouring an unknown poison into the springs supplying the rebelling cities. According to the Roman historian Florus (1.35.5–7), however, his victory brought dishonor to Rome because of the resort to underhanded biological tactics that also affected noncombatants. Two Carthaginian generals, Himilco and Maharbal, reportedly overcame enemies in North Africa by tainting wine with mandrake, a heavily narcotic root of the deadly nightshade [1].

In the first century BC, naturally occurring toxic honey was deployed against the army of the Roman general Pompey during the war against King Mithradates VI of Pontus on the southern coast of the Black Sea (northeastern Turkey). In 65 BC, Mithradates's allies gathered wild honeycombs, placed them along the Romans' route, and waited in ambush. In that region, wild bees gather nectar from profuse rhododendron blossoms; the honey does not harm the bees but contain devastating neurotoxins dangerous to animals and humans. The Roman legionnaires eagerly ate the sweet honey, and then they began collapsing with vertigo, vomiting, paralysis, and diarrhea. Mithradates's allies, who had been lying in ambush, came out and slaughtered 1000 of Pompey's men [1].

2.6 VENOMOUS INSECTS, SNAKES, AND SCORPIONS

Stinging insects such as wasps, deadly vipers, and scorpions could be enlisted as allies in war. Some scholars suggest that in Neolithic times, people threw hives filled with furious bees at enemies, who were thrown into chaos by the painful stings. Much later, in the Roman period, catapults were used to hurl beehives at foes. In Central Mexico, the ancient Mayans devised ingenious booby traps to repel besiegers on their fortress walls, consisting of dummy warriors with heads made of gourds filled with angry hornets [1,5].

In the Aegean off the coast of Turkey in the second century BC, the famous Carthaginian general Hannibal found himself outnumbered during a naval battle against Pergamon, which was ruled by Eumenes II. Hannibal ordered his men ashore to collect live vipers and pack them into clay pots. Then, as the enemy ships approached the Carthaginians vessels, Hannibal's men hurled the pots. As the catapulted pots smashed on the ships' decks, releasing masses of snakes, the Pergamene sailors panicked and were easily defeated [1].

A similar tactic using insects and arthropods saved the fortified city of Hatra (Iraq) in AD 198–199. Besieging Roman legions led by Emperor Septimius Severus were forced to retreat after the Hatreni defended their walls with terracotta pots filled with live scorpions, assassin bugs, and other poisonous insects from the surrounding desert. According to the Roman historian Herodian, as the insects rained down on the Romans scaling the walls, they "fell into the men's eyes and exposed parts of their bodies, digging in, biting, and stinging the soldiers, causing severe injuries." The terror effect would have been highly effective, no matter how many men were actually stung. Scorpion stings inject a complex combination of toxins, causing intense pain, thirst, great agitation, muscle spasms, convulsions, slow pulse, irregular breathing, and torturous death. Assassin bugs, large blood-sucking insects with sharp beaks, inflict an extremely painful bite and inject a lethal nerve poison that liquefies tissues. It is possible that Paederus rove beetles (*Staphylinidae*) were also collected in the desert by the defenders of Hatra. Pederin, the virulent poison secreted by predatory rove beetles, was well known in ancient India and China. Pederin is one of the most powerful animal toxins in the world, causing severe blistering of the skin and eyes. In the bloodstream, its toxicity is more potent than cobra venom [1].

2.7 AEROSOL AND INCENDIARY WEAPONS

Choking fogs and asphyxiating clouds of smoke, dust, and gases were effective chemical weapons in antiquity. One of the earliest documen-ted examples of toxic aerosols occurred during the Peloponnesian War in 429 BC. That year Sparta besieged the city of Plataia. The Greek his-torian Thucydides reported that the Spartans created a massive fire just outside Plataia's walls. The Spartans fueled the fire with great quantities of resinous pine tree sap (crude turpentine pitch) and sulfur. The combination of pitch and sulfur created great clouds of toxic sul-fur dioxide gas, fumes that can be fatal when inhaled in large amounts. A few years later, in 424 BC, the Boeotians, allies of the Spartans, invented a "flame throwing" machine. They used the contraption to propel billows of noxious smoke from charcoal, resin, and sulfur against the walled city of Delium.

Archaeologists have discovered physical evidence to show that in AD 256, the Sassanians attacking Roman-held Dura-Europos (on the modern border of Iraq and Syria) created a similar incendiary mixture of sulfur and pitch that resulted in a deadly gas enveloping a siege tunnel, suffocating 19 Romans and 1 Sassanian. The skeletons of 20 victims and residue of sulfur crystals and pitch burned in braziers to create poisonous sulfur dioxide gas were found in the tunnel [1,6].

Aeneas the Tactician, a Greek writing in 360 BC on how to defend against sieges, suggested the use of incendiaries made with pitch, hemp, and sulfur. Roman historians tell how burning chicken feathers created irritating, choking fumes that could be propelled by bellows into enemy siege tunnels.

In 80 BC in Spain, the Roman general Sertorius deployed choking clouds of dust to defeat the Characitani tribe, who had taken refuge in inaccessible limestone caves. The fine white soil around the cave formations consists of limestone and gypsum. Sertorius ordered his masked soldiers to sweep up great heaps of the powder in front of the caves. Then when the wind was just right, the Romans stirred up the dust with poles to raise great clouds of caustic lime powder, a severe irritant to the eyes and lungs. The Characitani surrendered (Plutarch, *Sertorius*). A similar choking tactic was used in China to quell an armed peasant revolt in AD 178, when "lime chariots" equipped with bellows blew limestone powder into the crowds. The powdered lime, which interacts with the moist membranes of the eyes, nose, and throat with corrosive, burning effect, blinded and suffocated the victims [1].

In the Middle East where crude petroleum is abundant, naphtha (the volatile and toxic light fraction of oil) was used as a weapon by itself and later, in the seventh century AD, perfected in Greek fire, whose exact recipe and delivery system have been lost [7,8]. Naphtha was ignited and poured on attackers with devastating effects (Pliny, *Natural History* 2.235). The ancient Indians and Chinese added combustible chemicals to their incendiaries, usually explosive saltpeter or nitrite salts, a key ingredient of gunpowder. The Chinese also used a variety of plant, animal, and mineral poisons, such as arsenic and lead, in making smoke and fire bombs even more harmful. In the New World and in India, the seeds of toxic plants and hot peppers were burned to rout attackers [1,2].

2.8 PRACTICAL ISSUES AND ETHICAL QUALMS

The toxicity of plants, venoms, and other poisons used in armaments often imperiled those who wielded them. Toxic weapons are notoriously difficult to control and often resulted in the destruction of noncombatants as well as soldiers, especially in siege situations. Both the ancient mythology and the ancient history of poison weapons abound with incidents of accidental self-injuries, friendly fire problems, and unintended collateral damage. Windborne toxins also incurred obvious "blowback" problems. Kautilya addressed this issue in his *Arthashastra*, and recommended that protective salves and other remedies be applied before deploying poisonous smokes [4].

The use of poisons in warfare led people to seek antidotes. Ancient Greek and Latin sources list hundreds of substances—from rust filings to poultices made from medicinal plants—that were thought to counteract specific weaponized poisons. Some believed that one could become invulnerable to toxins by ingesting minute amounts of various poisons over time. Mithradates VI of Pontus (d. 63 BC) was an early experimenter in creating a "universal antidote" of more than 50 poisons and antidotes in tiny amounts. It later became known as the Mithridatium. The recipe is lost but pills purporting to be the Mithradatium were ingested by every Roman emperor from Nero onward, and then by European royalty including Charlemagne and Henry VIII, in the hope of achieving immunity to poison [9].

Toxic weapons were surrounded by ambivalence in antiquity, even though there were few rules of war governing their use. In many cultures, the idea of weapons that delivered hidden poisons to make an enemy defenseless or experience excessive suffering aroused moral criticism. Nevertheless, their use was rationalized in many recorded instances. The ancient Greeks considered poisoned projectiles a cowardly weapon, for example, but their greatest mythic heroes, Hercules and Odysseus, resorted to such arms, and well poisonings and toxic aerosols were documented in historical Greek conflicts. Many Romans deplored poisoned arrows and poisoning water and food supplies (e.g., Tacitus, *Annals* 3.1; 5.2). Yet Roman generals occasionally turned to such strategies. In India, the Hindu *Laws of Manu* (dating to 500 BC) forbade the use of poisoned arrows (although it recommended spoiling the enemy's food and water). In the same era, Kautilya's *Arthashastra* extolled the advantages of poisoning projectiles, food, and water, and asphyxiating foes with chemical and disease-laden clouds of smoke. Notably, Kautilya stressed the deterrent effect of publicizing the horrid ingredients of one's toxic arsenal. That psychological strategy was apparently taken up by the Scythians and others who broadcast their recipes for poison arrows. In China, Sun Tzu's *Art of War* (500 BC) praised deceptive terror strategies based on fire, and other Chinese war treatises give recipes for making toxic aerosols and incendiaries. On the other hand, humanitarian codes of war in China (450–200 BC) forbade ruses of war and harming noncombatants [1,2,4].

A common rationale for the use of toxic weapons was self-defense. Besieged cities and desperate populations turned to biological weapons as a last resort, while some commanders resorted to poisons out of frustration, hoping to break stalemates or long sieges. Some situations—such as waging holy wars, quelling rebellions, and fighting people considered "barbarians" or somehow less than human—encouraged the indiscriminate use of unfair toxic weapons against entire populations. The threat of horrifying chemical or biological weapons could discourage potential invaders or bring quick capitulation. Some generals had no compunctions about using any weapons at hand. Some cultures considered poison arrows to be acceptable weapons in both hunting and warfare.

Human ingenuity in weaponizing natural forces in antiquity is impressive. Many ancient toxic weapons and tactics anticipated, in substance or principle, almost every basic form of biological and chemical weapon known today, from spreading plague to poisoning water. Asphyxiating clouds of smoke can be considered the precursors of mustard and other toxic gases first used in World War I. In the fourth century BC, the defenders of Tyre (Lebanon) catapulted red-hot sand onto Alexander the Great's men, causing gruesome deep burns and agonizing death. That weapon can be seen as the ancient prototype of the modern thermite bombs of World War II and white phosphorus bombs of the present day. The unquenchable burning, adhering effects of ancient petroleum-naphtha incendiaries anticipated the modern invention of napalm, so notorious during the Vietnam War. Today's advanced "calmative mists" and sedative-drugged water supplies, and the top-secret insect and animal-based weapons being developed by modern military scientists, also have antecedents in the ancient world [1].

Even the dangers of self-injury and the perilous problems of disposing of poison weapons were anticipated in antiquity. The ancient

Greek myth of the Hydra with its ever-proliferating heads with venom-dripping fangs is a fitting symbol of the dilemmas of creating toxic armaments. Hercules had to dispose somehow of the immortal central head of the Hydra, which could not be destroyed. His solution was to bury the eternally dangerous Hydra head deep underground, and he placed a huge boulder as a marker over the spot to warn people away. An analogous geological solution is used today to dispose of toxic and nuclear weapons. Their eternal, indestructible materials are to be buried deep underground in the deserts of New Mexico and other sites in the American West, necessitating warnings to future generations about the danger of the biochemical agents. Notably, a model for halting the proliferation of toxic weaponry is also found in Greek myth. The young archer who inherited Hercules' Hydra-venom arrows had experienced accidental grievous injury from the arrows himself before he deployed them against the Trojans. After the Trojan War, the old veteran decided to dedicate the terrible poison arrows in a temple of Apollo, the god of healing, rather than passing them on to the next generation of warriors [1].

REFERENCES

[1] Mayor A. Greek fire, poison arrows and scorpion bombs: biological and chemical warfare in the ancient world. New York, NY: Overlook Press; 2009.

[2] Sawyer R. The Tao of deception: unorthodox warfare in historic and modern China. New York, NY: Basic Books; 2007.

[3] Jones D. Poison arrows: North American Indian hunting and warfare. Austin, TX: University of Texas Press; 2007.

[4] Kautilya. Arthashastra [Rangarajan LN, Trans.]. Delhi: Penguin Classics; 1992.

[5] Lockwood J. Six-legged soldiers: using insects as weapons of war. Oxford: Oxford University Press; 2009.

[6] James S. Stratagems, combat, and "chemical warfare" in the siege mines of Dura-Europos. Am J Archaeol 2011;115:69–101.

[7] Forbes R. Bitumen and petroleum in antiquity. 2nd ed. Leiden: Brill; 1964.

[8] Partington J. A history of Greek fire and gunpowder. Baltimore, MD: Johns Hopkins University Press; 1999.

[9] Mayor A. The poison king: the life and legend of Mithradates, Rome's deadliest enemy. Princeton, NJ: Princeton University Press; 2010.

CHAPTER 3

Anthropogenic Air Pollution in Ancient Times

László Makra

3.1 POLLUTION OF THE ENVIRONMENT IN ANCIENT TIMES

Environmental pollution is coeval with the appearance of humans. When *homo sapiens* first made fire, the resulting smoke was, in effect, an early form of environmental pollution. The burning of fuels for heating and cooking has contributed to indoor air pollution. The walls of caves inhabited several thousands of years ago are covered with thick layers of soot. The presence of smoke in confined spaces must have made breathing difficult and irritated the eyes. In the few mummified bodies remaining from the Palaeolithic Era the lungs have a black tone. In the first inhabited areas, smoke was not driven away (one of the practical reasons might have been protection against mosquitoes) and the people dwelling in these inner areas found shelter in the smoke [1]. Millions of people continue to live this way today. In 1993, when we were in Nepal trekking in Langtang National Park, we visited many small villages and found accommodation at local houses on the southern slopes toward the High Himalayas. Even today, the smoke of fire is not driven away from the buildings. The walls of the houses are built of metamorphic slates with no bonding, and the roofs are covered with rush matting. When there is fire, it produces a thick smoke inside the house, irritating the eyes and making breathing difficult. It is impossible to sleep; one can only stay there for a short time. From the outside, the houses look as if they were on fire; smoke is streaming out through the slits and gaps of the walls. Humans seem to have been living together with this unhealthy form of air pollution for many thousands of years.

Indoor air pollution, especially particulate matter, was a significant problem in antiquity. Animal and vegetable oils were burned to provide light; furthermore, the houses were heated by wood and animal dung. All these materials produced high quantities of soot and toxic gases [2]. Capasso [3] examined skeletons buried by the volcanic eruptions of Vesuvius and found evidence of inflammation of the pulmonary tract.

History of Toxicology and Environmental Health. DOI: http://dx.doi.org/10.1016/B978-0-12-801506-3.00003-0

Histological assessment of the lungs of ancient human mummies has shown that anthracosis (accumulation of carbon in the lungs caused by inhaled smoke or coal dust) was a regular disorder in many ancient societies due to long exposure to the smoke of domestic fires. Smoke protected against mosquitoes and other insects; however, it greatly increased the risk of chronic respiratory diseases [2].

Environmental pollution was responsible for a variety of illnesses. The very first polluting material might have been human feces. Bowel bacteria living in the human body, such as *Escherichia coli*, might have easily gotten into the drinking water, infecting early humans. Even today, this type of environmental pollution causes illnesses affecting millions of people. In China, where a comprehensive system was developed for waste disposal, the use of human feces as a fertilizer was an important component of agricultural practice thousands of years ago. The high productivity of the alluvial plain in eastern China has been maintained in this manner for over 4000 years. This tradition is being followed today in several regions of China. As Han Suyin says, "In Chengtu (the capital of Szechuan Province) those families who owned the city sewers and this way could sell the accumulated feces in the countryside, belonged to the richest ones even in the twentieth century (till 1949)" [4]. The fertilization of rice paddies with feces contributed to the pollution of groundwater, making it unsuitable for drinking in all of tropical Asia. However, boiling the water results in the precipitation of salts, rendering it totally tasteless. The tradition of flavoring boiled water with tea leaves comes from China. It began spreading geographically about 2000 BC and ultimately spread throughout Asia [5].

Dust pollution also appeared in ancient times. Some of this was of natural origin, and Chinese and Korean writers have noted the easterly movement of yellow loess (sometimes called Kosa dust) for thousands of kilometers (e.g., [6]). According to Janssens, in the New Stone Age, people mining flint from the embedding limestone in the stone mines day after day might have suffered from silicosis, (see, for example, Obourg [4]). The all-day inhalation of dust was likely the underlying cause. Sometimes the geographical location of an area was responsible for the outbreak of certain diseases. Investigations revealed that near Broken, in the territory of recent Zambia, hominids that lived about 200,000 years ago suffered from lead poisoning. The reason for this illness was the transport of lead into the spring located next to the cave of a streak of ore [4].

The harmful activities of ancient civilizations caused long-lasting changes in the environment, the effects of which can be experienced even today. However, these effects appeared only regionally, not globally. Increasing soil alkalinity on the floodplains of the Tiger and Euphrates Rivers between 3500 BC and 1800 BC resulted in a gradual decrease of the productivity of Sumerian agriculture. Water used for irrigation raises the groundwater table, and if the extra water is not driven away by channels, soil becomes saturated with water, resulting in the dissolution of salts and their precipitation on the surface in the form of an impermeable layer. Sumerian people noted this process: "*the soil surface turned white.*" Water used for irrigation gradually made the region more and more unsuitable for agricultural production due to leaching of soil. This phenomenon largely contributed to the decline of the Sumerian culture. [4,7]. Babylonian and Assyrian law included clauses that discussed neighbors' property. Although the earliest laws, those of Hammurabi (twenty-third century BC), related mostly to water [8], smoke was typically treated in the same way in ancient law [9]. Around AD 200, the Hebrew *Mishnah* and its interpretation through the Jerusalem and Babylonian *Talmud* detailed pollution issues [10].

In ancient times, air pollution had substantial consequences only in the cities. The air of these early towns, as in some recent settlements, was filled with the penetrating smell of decaying organic domestic waste, rotting meat, and human feces. During a siege, when there was no chance to remove these waste materials, which emitted aggressive smells, unbearable conditions prevailed in settlements. According to Egyptian historical records, when Nubian troops encircled the city of Hermopolis, which is situated on the left bank of the Nile halfway between Theba and Memphis, the inhabitants surrendered, pleading for mercy, rather than bearing the putrid smell of their town's air [11]. In ancient cities, pollution deriving from unpleasant odors was an important concern. Aristotle (384−322 BC) proposed a rule in his work, *Athenaion Politeia*, according to which manure should be placed outside the town, at least 2 km away from the town walls [12]. Smoke stained marble in antique towns, giving it a grayish tone. This annoyed several classical poets as well (e.g., Horace (65 BC to AD 8) and motivated ancient Jews, among others, to introduce a list of laws [10]. In ancient times, smoke and soot represented the two major media of air pollution.

There are several examples of environmental pollution in China as well. Prior to the Tang era (618 AD—907 AD), the firs on the mountains of Shantung were logged and burned; later in the Tang era, the slopes of the Taihang mountains, located at the borderline of the Shansi and Hopei provinces, became barren [13]. Also at this time, dynasty forests were cut around Loyang, the capital, in a circle with a radius of 200 miles. The trunks of the trees were mostly used as firewood and partially burned to produce ink for governmental offices [14].

Urban air pollution, especially from the use of traditional fuels, depends on the dimensions of the given settlement and the extent of the built-up territory, as well as on the nature of the industrial activity. As urbanization progressed in China, in the Mediterranean Basin, and in northwestern Africa from about AD 1000, more and more people lived in smoky and sooty surroundings. Maimonides, the philosopher and physicist (1135—1204), who had comprehensive experience of the towns of that era from Cordoba to Cairo, found that urban air is "stuffy, smoky, polluted, obscure, and foggy." Furthermore, he thought that this condition is produced by "dullness preventing understanding, lack of intelligence, and amnesia" of the inhabitants [15].

On the other hand, traffic and transportation difficulties restricted the rate of air pollution within the cities. Industrial activities consuming the most energy (e.g., the production of tiles, glass, pottery, bricks, and cast iron) were located near the forests, since the transportation of fuels in large quantities to the cities would have been too expensive. This way, though air pollutants of industrial origin made the air smelly, only a few people inhaled it. Port cities were partial exceptions, as ships could transport wood and charcoal more economically. Hence, Venice could maintain its glass industry, ensuring its energy supply by the transportation of wood from distant places. However, the majority of urban air pollution derived from household fuels such as manure or wood but sometimes from smokeless charcoal as well [1]. The air of the Chinese cities might have been extremely polluted, too, because the developed water transport system (Big Channel) enabled the use of large quantities of fuel, at least in the Sung capital, Kaifeng. This city, 500 km south of Beijing, was probably the first one in the world to convert its energy supply from wood to coal. The transition occurred at the end of the eleventh century, when the city had about 1 million inhabitants. However, the coal-heating period was short, because Mongolian troops destroyed Kaifeng in 1126 and those who remained in the city died from plague in the early thirteenth century [16].

Intensive environmental pollution appeared simultaneously with the development of societies. Extensive environmental losses occurred even in the earliest societies. Air and water were polluted, soils were destroyed, and many animal and plant species were exterminated. However, environmental changes caused by the earliest societies were generally minor ones and followed by a rapid restoration of original conditions. Thanks to this, many people are not aware of the environmental losses triggered by the activities of early societies. Consequently, they tend to be more lenient toward these early societies than toward modern societies living in an urban environment. At the same time, there are examples of environmental activities in ancient times that resulted in long-lasting changes, the signs of which are observable even today. The cutting down of forests in large areas for building ships in ancient times might have contributed to the decrease of woodland coverage in the Balkan Peninsula, and in the territory of Greece. However, the drier summers and droughts in the Mediterranean might have contributed to this large-scale reduction of woodland areas as well [17]. Not that this latter fact has no relation to human activities. In Greece, due to the scarce summer precipitation, stunted plants and bushes develop that are suitable only for grazing of sheep and goats. These animals, by overgrazing the slopes of mountains, increase soil erosion. The thin soil layer that becomes loose is transported from the slopes by winter runoff, creating barren limestone surfaces quite rapidly as a final and complete stage of erosion.

There are several examples of deforestation in other regions as well. During the reign of King Solomon, cedar woodlands covered an area of 5000 km^2. Cedar woodlands were first mentioned in the literature between 2500 BC and 2300 BC. However, today very few cedars are found there. In the golden age of the Roman Empire, the whole main road from Baghdad to Damascus was shadowed by cedars. Today, the road between these cities is surrounded by desert [1].

Several cultures emphasize that one should live in harmony with the environment. However, even in those societies where this idea has been perpetually mentioned (e.g., in Asian societies), environmental ideas frequently lost out to financial demands.

Ancient Romans called air pollution *gravioris caeli* (heavy heaven) or *infamis aer* (infamous air) [2]. Air pollution problems of ancient times are mentioned even in the poems of classical poets. "The smoke, the wealth, the noise of Rome..." held no charms for the Roman poet Horace (65 BC–AD 8), who described the blackening of houses and temples by smoke [18]. He wrote that Roman buildings turned more and more dark from smoke and that this phenomenon might be observed in many other ancient cities as well. Seneca (4 BC–AD 65), the teacher of Emperor Nero (AD 37–68), was in poor health all his life, and his physician frequently advised him to leave Rome. In one of the letters he wrote to Lucilius in AD 61 he mentions that he must escape from the gloomy smoke and kitchen odors of Rome in order to get better [19].

Sextus Julius Frontinus (AD ~30–100), once governor of Britain, who later oversaw water supply to imperial Rome and wrote about it in his book *De Aquaeductu Urbis Romae*, believed his actions also improved Rome's air. Civil claims over smoke pollution were brought before Roman courts almost 2000 years ago [9]. According to the Roman law, cheese-making facilities should be established in such a way so that their smoke would not pollute other houses. Much similar material is available from the very important book *Pan's Travail* [20] and in Brimblecombe [21].

The Roman senate introduced a law about 2000 years ago according to which "Aerem corrumpere non licet" (polluting the air is not allowed). The *Institutes* issued under the Roman emperor Justinian in AD 535 were used as a text in law schools. Under the section "Law of Things," our right to the air is clear: "By the law of nature these things are common to mankind—the air, running water, the sea, and consequently the shores of the sea." (Lib. II, Tit. I: Et quidem naturali iure communia sunt omnium haec: aer et aqua profluens et mare et per hoc litora maris).

3.2 LEAD IN ANCIENT TIMES

3.2.1 Lead Mining and Exploitation

In the ancient Mediterranean, mining and metallurgy played a primary role in the economy. According to Xenophon (434–359 BC) and

Lucretius (98–55 BC), the smoke of lead mines in Attica was harmful to human health [22].

Lead is extracted from its most important ore, galena. The lead content of galena is 86.6%, but it also contains arsenic, tin, antimony, and silver. Most of the silver production in the world comes from galena and not from silver ore, since mining and exploitation of galena is much more significant. A long time after the introduction of silver coin as a currency (about 2700 BC), the primary aim of galena mining was to extract silver, and lead was considered to be only a by-product [23].

The oldest lead object found by archaeologists is a string of beads worn in Anatolia some 8000 years ago. Its use as jewellery suggests that this was a time when lead was still new and rare [24]. At the same time, lead mining started about 4000 BC. Considerable exploitation began about 1000 years later, when a new smelting technology was introduced in order to extract lead (and silver) from sulfide ores of lead. The exploitation of lead ores and use of lead became more and more important during the Copper, Bronze, and Iron Ages [25]. This progress was promoted by the introduction of silver coins and the development of Greek civilization. (During that time lead production was 300 times higher than that of silver.) Lead production reached its maximum of 80,000 metric tons/year—about the same magnitude as that of the Industrial Revolution some 2000 years later [26]—in the golden age of the Roman Empire. The most important lead mines were situated in the Iberian Peninsula, the Balkans, in the territory of ancient Greece, and in Asia Minor [25]. Lead production suddenly decreased after the fall of the Roman Empire and reached its minimum at about AD 900 with a mass of only some 1000 metric tons/year. Then production began to increase again, thanks to the new lead and silver mines opened in Central Europe after about AD 1000.

3.2.2 The Utilization of Lead

Lead mines during the Roman era were a plentiful source of the metal, as Pliny describes lead being found "in the surface stratum of the earth in such abundance that there is a law prohibiting the production of more than a certain amount" [27]. In Roman times, lead was the most popular metal and was widely used in everyday life. It has a number of useful properties that suit it to relatively low levels of technology. It melts at low temperatures, it is malleable and easy to work, it can be readily cast and joined, and it is resistant to corrosion. Thus it comes as no surprise that it found widespread application in the ancient world [28]. Its compounds were used as face powders, lipstick, and mask paint, as well as a coloring agent in paints. Furthermore, lead was used for preserving foods; it was even added to wine in order to prevent its fermentation. Lead compounds were used as a birth control medicine (for exterminating sperm) and as a kind of a spice, too. Cups, jugs, pots, and frying pans were made of lead alloys. Coins were also made of lead, as well as of alloys of lead with other metals such as copper, silver, and gold. Since it resists corrosion and can be processed easily, lead was extensively used in shipbuilding, house building, and for the construction of water pipes. During house building, hot lead poured between limestone/marble blocks served as a binder. In ancient Rome and in other cities of the Roman Empire, the construction of water pipes was the most important use of lead. Also, in Babylon, a water pipe made of lead was used for watering the hanging gardens built by King Nabu-kudurri-usur (Nebuchadnezzar) (605–562 BC). Because of the above-mentioned facts, lead is frequently referred to as a Roman metal [4,24].

3.2.3 Illnesses Caused by Lead

Both lead and its compounds are poisonous. Thanks to its relatively low volatility (lead vapour), as well as the volatility of some of its compounds [e.g., a petrol additive $(Pb(C_2H_5)_4)$] or solubility [e.g., $Pb(CH_3COO)_2$], it can easily get absorbed in the human body. Symptoms of lead poisoning are headache, nausea, diarrhea, fainting, and cramps.

Romans knew that lead was a dangerous metal, since they noticed the symptoms people who worked in lead mines suffered. Pliny wrote that "red-lead is a deadly poison and should not be used medicinally" and warned that the "exhalations from silver mines (i.e., galena mines) are dangerous to all animals" [27]. Furthermore, the geographer Strabo (3.2.8 C142) described (in about 7 BC) the high chimneys required to disperse the air pollutants during silver production in Spain. However, since lead was used extensively in everyday life, danger was taken out of consideration. Lead was believed to be less dangerous if it got into the body only in small doses. When carbon dioxide dissolved in water interacts with lead in the water pipes, it results in a possible enrichment of these dissolved lead compounds in the body; this process can easily lead to a so-called lead disease, a consequence of which might be paralysis. Ancient writers Xenophon and Lucretius observed the noxious emissions from metal mines of Greece, and Pliny declared that smelter emissions were dangerous to animals, especially dogs [29,30]. The presence of lead in food and drinking water might have led to infertility or stillbirth [31]. Nevertheless, mineworkers suffered the most from the harmful effects of lead. Hence, Romans generally made slaves work in mines. In Greco-Roman times, according to estimates, several hundred thousand people (mainly slaves) died of acute lead poisoning during the mining and smelting processes [25,26,32]. The credit for the first direct clinical account of lead poisoning has in recent times been accorded to Hippocrates [27].

The use of lead water systems represented a hazard to health, but both the Romans and the Greeks exposed themselves to a far greater risk. They found that coating their bronze or copper cooking pots with lead or lead alloys not only prevented leaching of copper from the pots, thus avoiding spoiling the taste of the food, but was also very useful in preparing wine and grape syrup (sapa), which was used almost exclusively as a sweetening agent. Pliny also advocated this dangerous practice. He writes, "Preference should be given to lead vessels... in boiling defrutum and sapa" [27]. One property of lead is inhibition of enzyme activity. Hence, sapa kept fruit from souring and fermenting and was used extensively as a preservative. In addition, sapa was found to improve the quality of a poor wine and to prolong the length of time for which any wine could be kept [27]. Adoption of the use of lead to sweeten wine in medieval Europe caused widespread illness [33].

Some authors contend the extreme behavior of Emperors Caligula (AD 12–41) and Nero might also have been the consequence of lead poisoning [31]. No aspect of the history of lead is likely to provoke as much interest and controversy as the prevalence of chronic lead disease (deriving from extensive lead mining and the wide-scale usage of devices made of lead) in antiquity and the suggestion that it played an important part in the decline of the Roman Empire [25,26,32]. On the other hand, there are some aspects on which this idea has been largely discredited. First, the lead-related gluttony and other excesses of the Julio-Claudian and Flavian emperors are difficult to reconcile with the loss of appetite and constipation that are among the prominent symptoms of chronic plumbism (lead poisoning). Second, the Empire attained its greatest wealth, power, and extent under Trajan and other effective emperors, who also consumed foods and drinks prepared in lead-made devices [28]. Third, most of the lead in the bones from citizens of Rome has come from postmortem absorption [34]. It is suggested that gradual depopulation was the main contributor to the failure of the Roman Empire, with lead-induced infertility possibly playing a lesser role [24]. The rise of Christianity might have also been a major reason [35]. The decline of the Roman Empire is a phenomenon of great complexity and it is too simple to ascribe it to a single cause.

3.2.4 Lead Pollution in Ancient Tooth Samples from the United Kingdom

English researchers, co-fellows of the Natural Environment Research Council and the British Geological Survey, studied the concentrations of lead in tooth enamels from Romano-British and early medieval people from various sites in the United Kingdom. Then, they compared the lead concentrations present in these people to that of their prehistoric forebears as well as that of the modern people living in the United Kingdom today. According to an extensive study on the tooth enamel lead concentration of adults living in the United Kingdom carried out in the early 1980s, the concentrations of lead displayed spatial variations with an average of 3 ppm. Some more recent analyses on modern children's teeth found lead concentrations with averages around a few tenths of ppm suggesting, as indicated also by the atmospheric data, that modern lead exposure is decreasing. On the other hand, Neolithic people living before the use of metals had tooth enamel lead concentrations that averaged around 0.3 ppm. These concentrations are only a tenth of the average for modern people and possibly similar to those in modern children.

When analyzing tooth enamels of Roman, Anglo-Saxon, and Viking people from the United Kingdom, researchers found individuals with tooth lead concentrations greater than 10 ppm, and occasionally even higher values. Concentrations of this magnitude among modern people can be associated with occupational or acute exposure, and suggests that lead pollution was a significant problem for both Romans and early medieval ancestors of British citizens.

The explanation may be that England, Scotland, Wales, and Ireland are all rich in natural lead deposits. Furthermore, each of these countries has abundant ores, which have been mined since antiquity. Probably, it was partly the richness of the country's lead ores, with their associated silver, of course, which led to Rome's initial interest in conquest of this most northerly reach of the Empire. It is also known that the Romano-British, Anglo-Saxon, and Viking people inhabiting the area of the United Kingdom were exposed predominantly to lead from ore sources, because of the characteristic isotopic composition of the lead remaining in their teeth.

On the other hand, high exposures were detected not only among people actively involved in lead mining, smelting, or metal working, but in the tooth enamels of children too. Thus high lead concentration was considered to be an environmental rather than occupational problem.

3.2.5 Lead Pollution on Regional and Hemispheric Scales

In 1957–1958, as part of the International Geophysical Year, the first extensive research programs were launched to analyze information stored in snow and ice layers of Greenland and the Antarctic that were hundreds of thousands of years old. The aim of this research was to establish a possible hemispheric scale of air pollution for a time period spanning many thousands of years. Later, the ice cores coming from this area served as substantial evidence of the atmospheric effects of human activities (e.g., [36–38]). In Greenland, the deepest boring corresponds to an interval of 7760 years, which is well before the time when silver was first smelted from galena. We can speak about background levels of the atmospheric lead concentration up to this period [23].

The chemical analysis of an ice core 9000 ft deep from Greenland (1 ft = 30.48 cm) enabled the collection of information on the atmospheric pollution for the past back to 7760 years. According to this, lead concentration in the atmosphere before the beginning of lead production, when atmospheric lead derived only from natural sources, was low. At this time, the enrichment factor of the atmospheric lead was near 1 (0.8), which indicated that this lead derived from soils and rocks. Three thousand years ago, the lead concentration of the atmosphere practically corresponded to the levels measured at the beginning of lead production. This means that anthropogenic lead emission was still negligible up to this time, considering the amount of lead that went into the atmosphere naturally. The atmospheric concentration of lead started to increase in the fifth century BC, and during Greco-Roman times (between 400 BC and AD 300), the enrichment factor of lead reached the value 4 and remained at the same high level for seven centuries. Four times higher lead concentration was detected for this period in the snow and ice layers of Greenland compared to the earlier, natural values. This is the earliest detected hemispheric-scale air pollution, dating almost 2000 years before the Industrial Revolution and well before any other polluting effect [26].

In the golden age of the Roman Empire, about 2000 years before, 5% of total processed lead (80,000 metric tons) got into the atmosphere, which might have resulted in an atmospheric emission peak of 4000 metric tons/year [26]. Regarding the economic development of the Roman Empire, Scheidel [39] associated the lead pollution level of the atmosphere with the annual number of shipwrecks (trade volume) and meat consumption (animal bones). Lead emission deriving from metal processing caused important local and regional air pollution all over Europe, which can be detected, e.g., in the lacustrine deposits of southern Sweden [40]. Furthermore, these emissions significantly polluted the troposphere over the Arctic [26].

Rosman examined the possible sources of lead pollution in the ancient atmosphere. According to the analysis of lead isotope ratios in ice cores, the mines in the territory of Spain proved to be the main sources of atmospheric lead. These mines were supervised by Carthage between 535 BC and 205 BC, and subsequently by the Romans till AD 410. About 70% of lead in the ice layers of Greenland from the period between 150 BC and AD 50 comes from the mines of Rio Tinto, in the southeastern part of Spain [41].

During the Greco-Roman age, an important part of the fourfold increase of lead concentration in the troposphere over Greenland came from lead/silver mining and processing. During the Roman Empire, 40% of the lead production in the world occurred in Spain, Central Europe, Britain, Greece, and Asia Minor [25]. Lead was smelted in open furnaces, for which the rate of emissions was not checked. The escaping small aerosol particles could have easily reached the Arctic region via routes that have become known only recently [26].

After the fall of the Roman Empire, atmospheric lead concentrations suddenly dropped to the background level that was characteristic 7760 years ago. In the medieval and Renaissance periods, it began to increase again, and 471 years before it reached a concentration double that detected during the Roman Empire [23]. In the seventeenth century, scientists identified widely illnesses in mining areas that were thought to arise from dispersion of the toxic elements [9]. Following the Industrial Revolution, the increase was continuous. From the 1930s till about 1960, snow and ice samples in Greenland indicated a rapid increase. This can be traced back to the antiknock additives of leaded fuels, which were used first in 1923 [29]. On a global scale, two-thirds of the leaded additives were used by the United States in the 1970s, 70% of which went directly into the atmosphere via exhaust gases of vehicles. Atmospheric lead concentrations measured in the 1960s were about 200 times higher than natural values. This is one of the most serious global-scale pollutions of the environment on the Earth ever recorded [23]. The sudden decrease observed after 1970 can be traced to an increasing use of unleaded fuels. In recent years, all petrol sold in the United States, and a gradually increasing ratio of that sold in Europe, has been unleaded [29]. Recently, Eurasia has been responsible for 75% of the atmospheric lead concentration on the Earth [41].

Lead pollution in the atmosphere has been detected over the Antarctic since the beginning of the twentieth century. The use of leaded fuels and then their cutback can also be detected. Furthermore, it can be established that an important part of anthropogenic lead comes from South America [23]. At the same time, natural concentration changes of lead (and other heavy metals) were also considerable over the Antarctic during the past ages. Low concentration values were detected in the Holocene period, while lead concentration was two orders of magnitude higher than this during the last glacial maximum, about 20,000 years ago [42].

3.3 COPPER IN ANCIENT TIMES

3.3.1 Copper Mining and Exploitation

Initially (about 7000 years ago), copper was produced from native copper. This was the main procedure for about 2000 years. Following this period, the discovery and introduction of a new smelting technique of oxide and carbonate ores as well as the appearance of tin-bronze brought the development of the real Bronze Age. From then on, production increased continuously. In the period 2700–4000 BP (before present), total production was about 500,000 metric tons [43,44].

Copper production suddenly increased in the Roman times. In this period, copper alloys were used more intensively and frequently, both for military and for civil purposes (e.g., minting). The production reached its maximum 2000 years ago with a mass of about 15,000 metric tons/year. In this period, the main copper mines were situated in the territory of Spain (half of total world production of the derived from the regions of Huelva and Rio Tinto) as well as in Cyprus and Central Europe [45]. Total production in the period 2250–1650 BP was about 5 million metric tons [46].

When speaking about any metals, peaks and decreases in production correspond to booms and busts of the production area. This statement is valid for both the Roman Empire and China. A decrease in mining of all metal ores, including copper, started with the weakening of the Roman Empire. After the fall of the Empire, copper production decreased significantly in Europe. World production stagnated at a mass of about 2000 metric tons/year until the eighteenth century and then started to increase again. This increase, from the European side, was especially attributable to the opening of new mines in the ninth century in the territory of Germany, and in the thirteenth century in Sweden (the latter particularly in the region of Falun) [47].

Outside the Roman Empire, important copper production occurred in Southwest Asia and the Far East. When the Han dynasty (206 BC– AD 220) extended its influence over Southwest Asia, copper production in China was about 800 metric tons/year. In the medieval age, most of the world's production came from China (during the rule of the northern Sung dynasty). In this period, Chinese production reached its maximum of 13,000 metric tons/year, and this resulted in peak world production of 15,000 metric tons/year in the AD 1080s. Most of the copper was used for minting [48]. During some hundred centuries after this period, production suddenly dropped to about 2000 metric tons/year in the fourteenth century), and increased again from the Industrial Revolution until recently. (As a comparison, world copper production was 10,000 metric tons/year at the beginning of the Industrial Revolution.) In Japan pollution from the extensive production of copper used in the manufacture of giant Buddhist statues gave rise to extensive environmental pollution starting in the eighth century [49].

3.3.2 Copper Pollution on Regional and Hemispheric Scales

Before the beginnings of anthropogenic use of copper, about 7000 years ago, all atmospheric copper derived from natural sources. This situation did not change until 2500 years ago. Since 2500 BP, atmospheric copper concentration has increased, which is a consequence of large-scale copper pollution in the northern hemisphere [50].

Copper emissions from ancient times to the recent period have been the results of mining and metallurgical activities. Other anthropogenic activities (e.g., the production of iron and nonferrous metals and wood burning) contribute to these emissions only to a lesser extent.

Emissions from copper production, in connection with a significant technological development, have considerably changed during the past 7000 years. In ancient times, due to the primitive smelting procedures, the emission factor was about 15% [44,45,50]. At the beginning, several steps of processing of sulfide ores (roasting, smelting, oxidation, and cleaning) were performed in open furnaces. Emission has been taken out of consideration until the Industrial Revolution. From that time onward, more sophisticated furnaces and more recent metallurgical procedures started to spread. In the middle of the nineteenth century, the processing procedure was reduced to five steps. These technological developments resulted in a significant decrease in the emission factor. In the twentieth century, this factor was only 1% and later, with the introduction of further modifications, it became a mere 0.25% [45,50].

Since Roman times, the Cu/Al ratio has increased in ice samples, which indicates that considerable copper pollution occurred in the troposphere over the Arctic in this period. This copper might have originated during the high-temperature phase of processing as small-sized aerosol particles, and then entered the atmosphere. These aerosols could easily reach the Arctic region from the middle latitudes where they originated (in Roman times, mainly the Mediterranean Basin, especially Spain; in the medieval period, China).

Changes of the Cu/Al ratio in the ice samples seem to correspond to estimated changes of anthropogenic copper emission. Data derived from ice cores from Greenland indicate low values until 2500 years before present, medium values from Roman times until the Industrial Revolution and suddenly increasing values near the recent period. Data from Roman times show high variability. This can probably be traced back to the fact that in this period the production of copper occurred over short periods and was dependent on how many copper coins were needed [50].

According to the ice samples from Greenland, when comparing production data with emission factors, atmospheric copper emission peaked twice in the period before the Industrial Revolution. The first peak occurred in the golden age of the Roman Empire, about 2000 years ago, with a mass of some 2300 metric tons/year, when the use of metal coins spread in the ancient Mediterranean. The second peak appeared in the golden age of the northern Sung dynasty in China (AD 960–1279), about AD 1080, with a mass of some 2100 metric tons/year, when the Chinese economy was extensively developing and copper production increased. Since the smelting technology was primitive at that time, about 15% of the smelted copper got into the atmosphere. Though the total copper emission of the Roman and Sung times was about a tenth of that in the 1990s, copper production did not reach even a hundredth of that in the recent period. Hemispheric copper pollution caused by copper emissions has a more-than-2500-year history and copper emissions of the Roman and Sung times were so high than never before the year 1750 AD [45].

3.4 ENVIRONMENTAL AWARENESS IN ANCIENT ISRAEL

The environment is a natural issue of concern in Judaism. Much of the discussions center on the Biblical commandment of *bal taschit*, i.e., not to destroy without purpose any object from which someone might derive pleasure. Trees, fields, and rivers belonged to this circle. Jewish people knew that trees were very important and, for this reason, they prohibited the cutting down of trees around cities. Furthermore, trees were required to be watered and the environment cared for. Any form of luxury was prohibited, because luxury itself is a kind of waste. Beyond the prohibition of actual destruction, an entire series of laws deals with maintaining the general environmental quality of life. The Talmud requires

1. that one must not open a shop in a courtyard if the noise pollution of customers will disturb the neighbors' sleep;

2. that one must put pigeon cotes at least 50 cubits from the town walls, so that the droppings will not damage the town's vegetable gardens;
3. that threshing floors must also be kept at this distance, to prevent the chaff from creating an air pollution problem for the city.

Carrion, graves, and tanneries had the same distance requirement because of the odors they produce.

The fifth book of Moses is the basis of Jewish ecology. It specified, among other things, that soldiers were prohibited to relieve themselves on the field of their camp. They were to leave the camp, dig a hole, and when they are finished, bury their output. It was prohibited to build a latrine near houses because latrines were malodorous. Since stench disseminates in a different way in winter than in summer, open sewer channels were prohibited during the summer. If anybody suffered from the sewage of another person, he or she could claim compensation. Sewage was not allowed to be released near kitchen gardens, because it decreased yields. Nature is natural and basic for Jewish people and they believe, even now, that one should live in the way that is prescribed in the Bible, Torah, and Talmud. The Biblical cities in Israel were surrounded by a *migrash*—an area of 1000 cubits left for public enjoyment in which nothing could intrude. For this reason, trees must be kept 25–50 cubits (depending on the species of tree and the amount of shade each species provides) from the city wall. Furthermore, according to the rabbis, the migrash may not be turned into a field, as that would destroy the beauty of the city. Interestingly, a field cannot be made into a migrash, as that will diminish crop production.

In temple services, olive wood and wood from grape vines are prohibited from use on the altar. One opinion is that this rule arose from concern for the settlement and cultivation of the land of Israel. The second opinion is much more specific. These types of woods burn with a great deal of smoke, and air pollution is to be avoided. Jerusalem, as the holiest of the cities, also had special environmental legislation designed to protect its unique environment for the enjoyment of its inhabitants and visitors. In that regard, all garbage was removed from the city, dunghills were prohibited from the city area, and no kilns were allowed to operate within its border. In this way, vermin and smoke were kept out of the city and the quality of life was improved [12]. Tanning facilities were to be placed at least 60 cubits from the city wall, because they were highly odoriferous. They were prescribed to be built on the eastern side of the city, since in Israel northerlies and westerlies were generally the most frequent winds; this way, the stench would not get back to the city. Mills had to be built at least 50 cubits from the city wall, because when they were operating much dust got into the air, which was harmful to humans when inhaled. Furthermore, it was said that wheat powder was not only unhealthy, but also harmful for the fields. Accordingly, mills should be built far away from fields. One can read in the Talmud that smoke is not only bad and harmful, but destroys the Garden of Eden of God as well. Hence, the relationship between God and humans becomes worse and they draw away from each other. The Talmud also says that the soul of God lives in everything: in animals, plants, and stones, etc. Therefore, He must not be offended, because if God had wanted a smoky world he would have created it. In the law-book of Tosefta, it was written that it was prohibited to wash in drinking water. Each well should be covered by a roof so that snakes, insects, and vicious souls could not to attack the water in it. Sewage holes were not allowed to be dug near a neighbor's well.

The Jewish law-books dealt with noise pollution, too. Millstones caused loud noise and vibration during work. For this reason, mills were not allowed to be established near the city. The operation of a school (if it was a big one with at least 50 students) depended on the inhabitants of the neighboring houses. Children caused lots of noise, and this could disturb the inhabitants [51].

This raises the question of why rabbis dealt so much with the environment in the past and why this environmental sensitivity was later pushed into the background. The answer might be that Jewish people didn't have farms for a long time, and thus didn't feel close to nature. Therefore, they didn't appreciate the value of a field as much as their ancestors did. Perhaps now that they can go back to their real homes, they will listen to the sounds of nature and their environment more carefully. According to the proverb, "The clean Jewish people take better care of their environment than the dirty Romans" [51].

ACKNOWLEDGMENT

The authors would like to express their gratitude to Claude F. Boutron (Laboratoire de Glaciologie et Géophysique de l'Environnement du Centre National de la Recherche

Scientifique, Unité de Formation et de Recherche de Mécanique Université Joseph Fourier, Grenoble, France) for his exceptionally comprehensive contribution, and Noa Feller, Ian Strachan, and Keith Boucher for their useful hints on the topic.

REFERENCES

[1] McNeill JR. Something new under the sun. An environmental history of the twentieth-century world. New York, London: W.W. Norton & Company; 2001.

[2] Colbeck I, Nasir ZA. Indoor air pollution. In: Lazaridis M, Colbeck I, editors. Human exposure to pollutants via dermal absorption and inhalation, 17. Dordrecht: Springer; 2010. p. 41–72.

[3] Capasso L. Indoor pollution and respiratory diseases in ancient Rome. Lancet 2000;356: 1774.

[4] Markham A. A brief history of pollution. London: Earthscan; 1994.

[5] Makra L. Wandering in China. Változó Világ 37. Budapest: Press Publica Kiadó; 2000 [in Hungarian].

[6] Chun Y. The yellow-sand phenomenon recorded in the Chosunwangjosilok. J Meteorol Soc Korea 2000;36:285–92.

[7] Mészáros E. The mankind and the environment before the industrial revolution. História 2002;5-6:21–4 [in Hungarian].

[8] Driver GR, Miles JC. The Babylonian laws legal commentary. Oxford: Clarendon Press; 1952.

[9] Brimblecombe P. The antiquity of smokeless zones. Atmos Environ 1987;21(11): 2485.

[10] Mamane Y. Air-pollution control in Israel during the 1st and 2nd century. Atmos Environ 1987;21(8):1861–3.

[11] Brimblecombe P. History of air pollution. In: Singh HB, editor. Composition, chemistry and climate of the atmosphere. New York, NY: Van Nostrand Reinhold; 1995. p. 1–18.

[12] Mészáros E. A short history of the Earth. Budapest: Vince Publisher Ltd; 2001 [in Hungarian].

[13] Schäfer EH. The conservation of nature under the tang dynasty. J Econ Soc Hist Orient 1962;5:299–300.

[14] Epstein R. Pollution and the environment. Vajra Bodhi Sea: A Monthly Journal of Orthodox Buddhism 1992;Pt. 1, v. 30:36, 12.

[15] Turco RP. Earth and seige: from air pollution to global change. Oxford: Oxford University Press; 1997.

[16] Hartwell R. A cycle of economic change in imperial China: Coal and Iron in Northeast China, 750–1350. J Econ Soc Hist Orient/Journal d'Histoire economique et sociale de l'Orient 1967;10:102–59.

[17] Karatzas K. Preservation of environmental characteristics as witnessed in classic and modern literature: the case of Greece. Sci Total Environ 2000;257:213–8.

[18] Costa CDN. Dialogues and letters: Seneca. London: Penguin Books; 1997.

[19] Heidorn KC. A chronology of important events in the history of air pollution meteorology to 1970. B Am Meteorol Soc 1978;59:1589–97.

[20] Hughes JD. Pan's Travail. Baltimore: John Hopkins University Press; 1993.

[21] Brimblecombe P. The big smoke. A history of air pollution in London since medieval times. London, New York: Methuen; 1987.

[22] Weeber KW. Smog über attika: umveltverhalten im altertum. Artemis. Zürich; 1990.

[23] Boutron CF. Historical reconstruction of the Earth's past atmospheric environment from Greenland and Antarctic snow and ice cores. Environmental Rev 1995;3:1–28.

[24] Eisinger J. Lead in history and history of lead. Nature 1984;307(5951): 573.

[25] Nriagu JO. Lead and lead poisoning in antiquity. New York, NY: Wiley; 1983.

[26] Hong S, Candelon JP, Patterson CC, Boutron CF. Greenland ice evidence of hemispheric lead pollution two millennia ago by Greek and Roman civilizations. Science 1994;265:1841–3.

[27] Waldron HA. Lead poisoning in the ancient world. Med Hist 1973;17:391–9.

[28] Waldron HA. Medical History 29(1). Cambridge: Cambridge University Press; 1985. p. 107 – 108. doi:10.1017/S0025727300043878.

[29] Nriagu JO. Global metal pollution: poisoning the biosphere. Environment 1990;32(7):8.

[30] Morin BJ. Reflection, refraction, and rejection: copper smelting heritage and the execution of environmental policy (PhD dissertation). Michigan Technological University; 2009.

[31] Goldstein E, editor. Pollution. Boca Raton, FL: Social Issues Resources Series, Inc; 1988.

[32] Nriagu JO. Occupational exposure to lead in ancient times. Sci Total Environ 1983;31:105–16.

[33] Eisinger J. Early consumer protection legislation—a 17th C law prohibiting lead adulteration of wines. Interdiscipl Sci Rev 1991;16:61–8.

[34] Fouache E. Using the geo-archaeological approach to explain past urban hazards. In: Serre D, Barroca B, Laganier R, editors. Resilience and urban risk management. London: Taylor & Francis Group; 2013. p. 15–20.

[35] Zeek WC. Technology and culture. In: Nriagu JO, editor. Lead and lead poisoning in antiquity, New York: Wiley & Sons; 1983. p. 129–30.

[36] Boutron CF, Görlach U, Candelone JP, Bolshov MA, Delmas RJ. Decrease in anthropogenic lead, cadmium and zinc in Greenland snows since the late 1960s. Nature 1991;353:153–6.

[37] Boutron CF, Rudniev SN, Bolshov MA, Koloshnikov VG, Patterson CC, Barkov NI. Changes in cadmium concentrations in Antarctic ice and snow during the past 155,000 years. Earth Planet Sci Lett 1993;117:431–44.

[38] Boutron CF, Candelone JP, Hong S. Past and recent changes in the large scale tropospheric cycles of Pb and other heavy metals as documented in Antarctic and Greenland snow and ice: a review. Geochim Cosmochim Ac 1994;58:3217–25.

[39] Scheidel W. In search of Roman economic growth. J. Roman Archaeol 2009;22(1):46–70.

[40] Renberg I, Persson MW, Emteryd O. Pre-industrial atmospheric lead contamination detected in Swedish lake sediments. Nature 1994;368:323–6.

[41] Rosman KJR, Chisholm W, Boutron CF, Candelone JP, Görlach U. Isotopic evidence for the sources of lead in Greenland snows since the late 1960s. Nature 1993;362:333–5.

[42] Boutron CF, Patterson CC. Lead concentration changes in Antarctic ice during the Wisconsin/Holocene transition. Nature 1986;323:222–5.

[43] Tylecote RF. A history of metallurgy. London: Mid-County; 1976.

[44] Morin BJ. The legacy of American copper smelting: industrial heritage versus environmental policy. Knoxville, TN: University of Tennessee Press; 2013.

[45] Hong S, Candelone JP, Soutif M, Boutron CF. A reconstruction of changes in copper production and copper emissions to the atmosphere during the past 7000 years. The Sci Total Environ 1996;188:183–93.

[46] Healy JF. Mining and metallurgy in the Greek and Roman world. London: Thames and Hudson; 1988.

[47] Pounds NJG. An historical geography of Europe. Cambridge, London: Cambridge University Press; 1990.

[48] Archaometallurgy Group. Beijing university of iron and steel technology. Beijing: A Brief History of Metallurgy in China. Science Press; 1978.

[49] Satake K. New eyes for looking back to the past and thinking of the future. Water Air Soil Poll 2001;130(1-4):31–42.

[50] Hong S, Candelone JP, Patterson CC, Boutron CF. History of ancient copper smelting pollution during Roman and medieval times recorded in Greenland ice. Science 1996;272:246–9.

[51] Schwartz E. Bal Tashchit: A jewish environmental precept. In: Yaffe MD, editor. Judaism and Environmental Ethics: A Reader. Lanham, Md: Lexington Books; 2001.

CHAPTER 4

Poisoning in Ancient Rome: The Legal Framework, The Nature of Poisons, and Gender Stereotypes[1]

Evelyn Höbenreich and Giunio Rizzelli

4.1 *VENEFICIUM* AND LEGAL TERMINOLOGY

For the Romans, poisoning (*veneficium*) was a crime committed by administering *venena*, which referred to substances or practices that may also belong to the sphere of magic and can alter anything they come into contact with (including both a person's body and mental state). The act of using *venena* is considered to be a *veneficium*, penalized, and, accordingly, punished, if—dependent on the period and the context—the effects caused by the *venena* are deemed harmful or censurable from an ethical point of view. A law dating from the age of Sulla was the *lex Cornelia de sicariis et veneficis*. This law, passed in 81 BCE, not only contained provisions against persons intent on killing or stealing (*sicarii*), but also persecuted the *venefici*, the perpetrators of *veneficium*, an activity which consisted of the preparation or administration of *venena*. According to Cicero (*Cluent.* 148), the fifth chapter of the *lex Cornelia* ordered the punishment of anyone who prepared, sold, bought, kept, or administered a noxious poison (*venenum malum*). It almost seems as if the Sullan law had enumerated the single criminal activities in the chronological order in which they succeed each other: the preparation, selling, acquisition (hence possession), and, eventually, the administration of the substance for the purpose of killing.

The legal literature confirms the reference found in the speech of Cicero in defence of Cluentius. Indeed, similar references are found in the work of the jurist Marcianus at the beginning of the third century CE, and in a later legal text, the so-called *Pauli sententiae* (PS.). Marcian. 14 *inst.* D. 48.8.1.1, states. "Someone is also liable who

---

[1]The ancient Greek and Latin sources have been translated into English by the authors of this article. For the translation of the text from Italian into English we are obliged to Sebastian Puchas and Marlene Peinhopf. We thank Aglaia McClintock for checking the abstract.

History of Toxicology and Environmental Health. DOI: http://dx.doi.org/10.1016/B978-0-12-801506-3.00004-2

formulates <and> administers poison for the purpose of killing a man." In Marcian. 14 *inst*. D. 48.8.3 pr.1 can be read. "Under chapter five of the same *lex Cornelia*, focusing on armed 'gangsters' or murderers and poisoners, anyone is punished who makes, sells, or possesses a drug (*venenum*) for the purpose of homicide. § 1. The person who sells harmful medicines (*mala medicamenta*) to the public or possesses them for the purpose of homicide is liable to the penalty of the same law." And, eventually, PS. 5.23.1: "The *lex Cornelia* imposes the penalty of deportation on a person who has kept, sold, or prepared a poison (*venenum*) in order to procure the death of a man."

Although Cicero's and Marcianus's descriptions are not in agreement on every point, both concur with the assessment of *venenum* as *malum* (noxious or harmful). The assessment of the *venenum* as "harmful" in the Ciceronian text concurs with the description found in the Marcianian text, which asserts that the penalized behavior is calculated to cause the death of a (hu)man. Although the formulations of Cicero and Marcianus do not coincide on every point, both indicate that a certain behavior comes within the scope of criminal law, if the preparation, possession and administration of *venenum* is aimed at killing somebody. Furthermore, the jurist also attests to an extension of the law so that the punishment inflicted on both those who sell lethal substances to the public and those who keep substances that could be used to cure (what one might refer to as drugs nowadays), with the intention to kill, is the same as that outlined in the *lex Cornelia* with reference to the *sicarii* and *venefici*. Marcianus, however, does not actually use the term *malum* with regard to *venenum*, because that adjective is reserved for *medicamenta* (*mala medicamenta*), indicating that the substances or concoctions aimed at healing somebody could also have lethal effects: If intention to kill by their use is proved, their possession is punished; if murder is not the intention, but the person who has consumed the substance perishes nonetheless, the seller of the substance is still punished.

4.2 PERPETRATORS, TRIALS, STEREOTYPES

In the historical sources, the charge of poisoning is frequently brought against women. Cases typically concern a woman of low social status whose profession is preparing *venena*. Among these women is Locusta, who provided the poison Agrippina used to kill Claudius or Nero to murder Britannicus. Tacitus (*ann.* 12.66 and 13.15) mentions her as notorious for her many crimes. The charge of poisoning, however, can also concern persons of higher status, even the empress Livia Drusilla, wife of Augustus; she was suspected, rightly or wrongly, of being responsible for the deaths of Marcellus, Gaius, Lucius, and even the *princeps* Augustus himself, in order to assure the succession of her son, Tiberius Claudius Nero (cf. Tac. *ann.* 1.3 and 5; Cass. Dio 53.33.4, 55.10a.8-10). These passages make no explicit reference to the act of poisoning, but the descriptions of the crimes allow one to extrapolate to this conclusion with reasonable certainty.

For a long time the notion of *veneficium* continued to be related to magic; consequently, the woman concocting or administering the poison was regarded somehow as a sorceress. By the way, it had been widely accepted that the female universe was strongly bound to the magical sphere, particularly regarding seducing and "bewitching" a man. A famous case in point can be found in the passage in which Cassius Dio depicts how Cleopatra reduced Mark Antony to her slave by availing herself properly of those arts, combined with her *eros* (Cass. Dio 49.33.4).

Long before the *lex Cornelia de sicariis et veneficis*, a trial took place before the *comitia* (one of the people's assemblies operating mostly during the time of the Republic before which also criminal proceedings took place) in 331 BCE and concluded with the conviction of 170 matrons. The short account written by Valerius Maximus (2.5.3) at the beginning of the Principate (i.e., the time from Augustus to the Severan Emperors; the death of Alexander Severus in 235 CE also marked the end of a flourishing jurisprudence) shows that the case was seminal in that it led to a series of trials involving various acts considered to be cases of *veneficium*.

As Maximus explains, the victims of these crimes were the husbands of the female perpetrators. Using poison, they killed by stealth, that is, in what was considered an insidious and detestable way, since self-defense typically was not possible. Crimes of this nature were thought to be particular to weak people, incapable of confronting their opponents openly and directly. Indeed, that which in this passage is present only as a faint echo is commonplace in Greek and Latin literature, which is rooted in the cultural representation of the female physiology and psychology—the weakness of the former alludes to the fragility of the latter. As expounded in a short treatise on physiognomy which the ancients attributed to Aristotle (and which, at any rate, perfectly fits into the Peripatetic tradition), female animals, being less strong and courageous than their male counterparts, are therefore all the more insidious (i.e., there is said to be a strong connection between weakness, cowardice, and a disposition to injustice: *Physiogn.* 809a. 26-810a. 8). This treatise, in suggesting that the occult nature of poisoning and its evil intention may be due to women's weak nature, thus aligns with Maximus' observations.

Over the centuries, this motive does not seem to have lost any of its strength. For example, at the end of the nineteenth century an Italian forensic physician named Giuseppe Ziino pointed to it to comment on a statistic showing that more females than males were among the accused, and to explain that "the innate weakness of women, even more than their perfidiousness, induces them to use a weapon which kills insidiously and does not force the (female) murderer to fight openly with the victim." The topic is also a subject of discussion by other famous authors, including Cesare Lombroso and Richard von Krafft-Ebing, where instead of scientific arguments we encounter the proverb or the commonplace. Thus, in an influential physiological-criminological manual written by Gustav Aschaffenburg for physicians, jurists, and sociologists in 1902 and dedicated to the celebrated psychiatrist Emil Kräpelin, one reads: "All in all, the female crime is characterized rather by baseness, the male crime rather by brutality."

4.3 TRAINING FOR THE COURTS

These incidents hardly exhaust the cases of *veneficium* committed by women against their husbands. There is, however, according to the ancient sources, another reason attributed to women's predilection for poisoning—that of their insatiable erotic desire, impelling them to commit *veneficium* in connection with adultery, which basically can also be described as a kind of *veneficium*. The adulteress commits this *veneficium*, one might say, by engorging herself with the fluid of a male to whom she is not married.

The strong connection between adultery and poisoning, for which women are held responsible as perpetrators, emerges by a striking example of *ratiocinatio*—that is, reasoning by posing a statement, questioning the statement, and answering the question. This device may be found in a compendium of rhetoric compiled in the first decades of the first century BCE, known as the *Rhetorica ad Herennium* (*Rhet. Her.* 4.23): "When our ancestors condemned a woman for one crime, they considered that by this single judgment she was convicted of many transgressions. How so? Judged unchaste, she was also deemed guilty of poisoning. Why? Because, having sold her body to the basest passion, she had to live in fear of many persons. Who are these? Her husband, her parents, and the others involved, as she sees, in the infamy of her dishonor. And what then? Those whom she fears so much she would inevitably wish to destroy. Why inevitably? Because no honorable motive can restrain a woman who is terrified by the enormity of her crime, emboldened by her lawlessness, and made heedless by the nature of her sex. Well now, what did they think of a woman found guilty of poisoning? That she was necessarily also unchaste. Why? Because no motive could more easily have led her to this crime than base love and unbridled lust. Furthermore, if a woman's soul had been corrupted, they did not consider her body chaste. Now then, did they observe this same principle with respect to men? Not at all. And why? Because men are driven to each separate crime by a different passion, whereas a woman is led into all crimes by one sole passion." This is what a young contemporary Roman who was preparing to embark on a forensic career learned.

The stereotype of the adulteress-*venefica*-sorceress also assumes concrete characteristics in some women accused in famous trials held at the beginning of the Principate. Thus, during the reign of Tiberius, among the charges brought against Lepida (she was sentenced for having simulated a birth with the intention of giving her husband a false heir), are accusations of adultery and *veneficium*. She is also accused of having consulted Chaldean astrologers as to the destiny of the imperial family (Tac. *ann.* 3.22-23). Claudia Pulchra, to give another example, is persecuted for having committed adultery and *veneficia* against the *princeps*, and for having performed *devotiones*, or magical arts (Tac. *ann.* 4.52.1 and 3).

Of course, men also commit poisoning, as the ancient authors confirm in abundance, but nonetheless, women are the primary perpetrators of this crime. Such a fact is observed by Quintilian in his work on the training of orators, where he deals with probative arguments, and their origins, like the sex of the perpetrator. Indeed, as an example he asserts that it was easier to believe that an act of banditry (*latrocinium*) was committed by a man and that an act of *veneficium* was the work of a woman (Quint. *inst.* 5.10.24). It is again Quintilian who returns to the argument of the adulteress who kills by poison. In a reference to the authority of wise men and famous citizens as particularly efficient witnesses, he quotes a sentence by Cato (Quint. *inst.* 5.11.39): "If an adulteress is on her trial for poisoning, is she not already to be regarded as condemned by the judgment of Marcus Cato, who asserted that every adulteress was as good as a poisoner?" Indeed, the orators elaborate this motive by investigating its different outcomes in various Latin declamations (exercises which were considered indispensable for those who, between the end of the Republic and the first years of the Principate, decided to dedicate themselves to the art of forensic oratory) that have come down to us.

4.4 JURISTS AND THE INTERPRETATION OF LAWS

Even if poisoning was not intentional, it was nevertheless often caused by females. This is recorded in the jurisprudential literature that deals with situations arising in connection with the storage, handling, and provision of *venena*. Marcianus (14 *inst.* D. 48.8.3.2) mentions a decree of the Senate (*senatus consultum*), probably dating from the first century CE, in which a woman was found guilty of having administered a medication to another woman in order to facilitate her conception of a child (the jurist speaks of a drug *ad conceptionem*); instead, the medication caused her death. The woman who administered the drug was found guilty by the Senate and in the sentence concluding the trial was condemned to relegation (a form of banishment to or from a certain place).

The Senate had punished the woman because she had administered a drug that caused the death of a person. Although the Senate probably wanted to make a clear statement against practices deemed to be socially dangerous, this punishment, according to Marcianus, was based on the fact that the action was considered a "bad example" and not because it was aimed at killing the woman who took the medication. Therefore, it went beyond the original scope of Sulla's law, which contained provisions against all who made, sold, bought, kept, or administered poison for the purpose of killing.

For a full understanding of the jurist's discourse, it is necessary to remember what else Marcianus stated immediately prior to that: namely, that for the *lex Cornelia* to be applied, the concocted potion must be qualified as *venenum malum*. In the case in question, the medication is not considered *malum*—that is, harmful and aimed at causing death. This point clearly emerges from the fact that, as Marcianus argues, *venenum* is a neutral designation that may refer either to substances for the purpose of healing or to those for the purpose of killing. As the jurist points out, the *amatorium* (the aphrodisiac draught), another commonly used drug, is also considered to be a *venenum*. This notion is confirmed by another *senatus consultum* mentioned in the subsequent paragraph of the same fragment. The Senatorial statute extended the *lex Cornelia* to the careless administration (which, therefore, probably, had caused some harm) of substances like the mandragora and the salamander, which were also known for being aphrodisiacs, by dealers in cosmetics, spices and unguents—the *pigmentarii*.

The *senatus consultum*, as can be read in Marcianus's fragment (14 *inst.* D. 48.8.3.3), supplements and generalizes the provision in § 2 by extending the penalty of the *lex Cornelia* to the careless (*temere*) administration of substances, which in principle can cure but which, owing to their potential toxicity, may also have harmful effects. The jurist's enumeration is not to be seen as exhaustive: "It is laid down by another *senatus consultum* that dealers in cosmetics, spices and unguents are liable to the penalty of this law if they recklessly hand over to anyone hemlock (*cicuta*), salamander (*salamandra*), monkshood (*aconitum*), pinegrubs (*pituocampis*), a beetle (*buprestis*), mandragora (*mandragora*), Spanish fly (*cantharis*) and whatever is prepared to cure a person" (Marcian. 14 *inst.* D. 48.8.3.3). As all of the mentioned substances can be used as medicines as well as poison (some also as aphrodisiacs), and their administration is punished only if done carelessly, it must be presumed that they have been given as *venena bona*, that is, for therapeutic purposes. However, if the substance is not administered with the intent to kill, how can one determine whether it was given carelessly? The answer is as follows: only if it has lethal consequences or causes somebody's health to decline considerably.

Marcianus observes that, apart from harmful *venena*, other *venena* exist that are not harmful (which serves to explain why one may be liable for preparing or administering a drug without the premeditated harmful consequences). This observation is confirmed by Roman legal literature, in an explanation by Gaius, at some prior time, in his commentary on the XII Tables (4 *ad l. XII tab.* D. 50.16.236pr.).

The *venenum*, explains the jurist, must be qualified as either "inoffensive" (*bonum*) or "harmful" (*malum*), because the term *venena* (drugs) embraces also *medicamenta* (medical substances, medicaments). Gaius continues that '*venenum*' is, in general, a substance capable of changing the nature of whatever it comes into contact with. Similarly, he notes, in the Greek language, *phármakon* refers to both substances that may cure and substances that may harm, thus to both medications and poisons. In order to support his own argument, Gaius calls to witness a very respectable source, namely a Homeric verse (*Od.* 4.230) taken from the description of the drugs Helen was taught to prepare by the Egyptian woman Polydamas, who hailed from a country where a great variety of such substances were produced. The double function of the *phármaka* may indeed be a motive that, in the period in which Gaius wrote, apparently had been popular in Greek literature for centuries. An example is to be found precisely in connection with Helen, in the *Encomium*, written toward the end of the fifth century BCE by the sophist Gorgias of Leontini. The author, perhaps referring to the medical knowledge of the time, distinguishes among *phármaka* that cure and *phármaka* that kill (§ 14).

The jurists' efforts to define the notion of *venenum*, which is important for the purpose of the *lex Cornelia de veneficis*, are justified by the circumstance that an obvious connection exists between the nature of the substance in question and the criminal intent of the person who intends to commit *veneficium*. The intent of the perpetrator seems to be more obvious if the substance in question is a poison, that is, a *venenum malum*. On the other hand, one and the same *venenum* may be used for different purposes, be they legal (aimed at healing) or illegal (aimed at impairing health or killing), depending on the dose, method of administration, and the like. The mandragora, for example, can be used as a sleeping aid but, if consumed in an abusive way, it may also have lethal consequences.

This double function of the *venena* presents the orators with an opportunity to invoke rather sophisticated arguments. These arguments illustrate how a substance meant to cure can have lethal effects or how what is normally considered a poison can have healing effects. In a borderline case, the consumption of icy water caused the death of the person to whom it was administered. Thus it seems obvious that the perpetrator's intent to kill, as well as facts beyond simply proving possession of *venenum*, had to be proved in order to reach a ruling.

The legal thought was that it was necessary to limit the spread of life-threatening practices by prosecuting the use of *venena* of any kind, which, even though the defendant was innocent of malicious intention, culminated in lethal effects. Such a hypothesis would have to be extrapolated from the original wording of the Cornelian law.

In any case, the legal provisions relating to the careless administration of certain medications, as described in the fragment by Marcianus, have been subjected to several modifications in the course of time. At least that is the case with an *amatorium*. Administration of aphrodisiacs and birth control agents have been penalized over time, even if they did not cause the death of the person consuming the drugs, simply because it was considered setting a "bad example." This determination is confirmed in the *Pauli sententiae* (PS. 5.23.145 = Paul. 5 *sent*. D. 48.19.38.5): "Those who administer an abortifacient or aphrodisiac draught, even if they don't do it with bad intention, are still condemned to the mines, if of lower rank, or relegated to an island with the forfeiture of part of their property, if of higher status, because the deed sets a bad example. But if for that reason a man or woman died, they are punished with a horrific form of death."

Thus, in this case—unlike what occurred at the time of Marcianus— the mere administration of abortifacients and aphrodisiac draughts was subject to penalty, even if it did not cause the death of anyone, because such activities were considered *mali exempli res*. The punishment that was imposed varied, depending on whether the perpetrators were persons of lower rank (*humiliores*) or of higher position (*honestiores*)—categories that were very prominent in the *Pauli sententiae*. If in consequence of such an administration of poison someone died, the perpetrator was subjected to the *summum supplicium* (i.e., the most atrocious form of death penalty). It is unknown whether this also applied to fertility drugs, *ad conceptionem*, which are mentioned by the Severan jurist. The precise reference to the abortifacient or the *amatorium* may indicate that the pseudo-Paulinian text was inspired by a legal provision concerning a particular case (although it may simply be that abortifacient and aphrodisiac draughts are mentioned only as examples). At any rate, the passage seems to justify a legal policy that offers severe responses to those who were professionally preparing and dealing with hazardous drugs and unguents.

We must not forget, however, that in the background of these texts, which are so important for reconstructing the legal practices of ancient

Rome, we may observe the ghosts conjured up by the poets. These images of poisoning have given rise to fears and anxieties that have haunted society's collective imagination for centuries. They call up visions of the tragic figure of Phaedra, whom Propertius (2.1.51-54) tells us devoted herself in vain to preparing potions that would make her stepson fall in love with her, or that of Medea, a passionate woman, but also a dangerous sorceress, furious and fatal in her quest for revenge.

SELECTED BIBLIOGRAPHY

Aschaffenburg G. Das Verbrechen und seine Bekämpfung. Einleitung in die Kriminalpsychologie für Mediziner, Juristen und Soziologen; ein Beitrag zur Reform der Strafgesetzgebung. 3. Aufl C. Winter, Heidelberg; 1923.

Cavaggioni F. *Mulier rea. Dinamiche politico-sociali nei processi a donne nella Roma repubblicana.* Venezia: Istituto Veneto di Scienze, Lettere ed Arti; 2004.

Cherubini L. *Strix. La strega nella cultura romana.* Torino: UTET Libreria; 2010.

Cloud JD. The primary purpose of the *Lex Cornelia de sicariis et veneficis.* Zeitschrift der Savigny-Stiftung für Rechtsgeschichte. Romanistische Abteilung (ZSS.RA) 1969;86:260−83.

Cloud JD. *Leges de sicariis:* The first chapter of Sulla's *lex de sicariis.* Zeitschrift der Savigny-Stiftung für Rechtsgeschichte. Romanistische Abteilung (ZSS.RA) 2009;126:114−55.

Ferrary J-L. Lex Cornelia de sicariis et veneficis. Athenaeum 1991;79:417−34.

Höbenreich E. Due senatoconsulti in tema di veneficio (Marcian. 14 inst. D. 48.8.3,2 e 3). Archivio Giuridico "Filippo Serafini" (AG) 1988;208:75−97.

Höbenreich E. Überlegungen zur Verfolgung unbeabsichtigter Tötungen von Sulla bis Hadrian. Zeitschrift der Savigny-Stiftung für Rechtsgeschichte. Romanistische Abteilung (ZSS.RA) 1990;107:249−314.

Kaufman DB. Poisons and poisoning among the Romans. Class Philol 1932;27:161−4.

Lombroso C, Ferrero W. The female offender. New York: D. Appleton & Co.; 1895.

Nardi E. Il procurato aborto nel mondo greco romano. Milano: Giuffrè; 1971.

Nörr D. *Causa mortis. Auf den Spuren einer Redewendung.* München: C.H. Beck; 1986.

Redl G. Die fahrlässige Tötung durch Verabreichung schädigender Substanzen im römischen Strafrecht der Prinzipatszeit. Revue Internationale des Droits de l'Antiquité (RIDA) 2005;52:309−24.

Rizzelli G. In: Rodríguez López R, Bravo Bosch MJ, editors. Note sul *veneficium. Mulier. Algunas Historias e Instituciones de Derecho Romano.* Madrid: Editorial Dykinson; 2013. p. 1−20.

Roman Statutes. In: Crawford MH, editor. Institute of Classical Studies, School of Advanced Study, Vol. II. London: University of London; 1996.

von Krafft-Ebing R. *Psychopathia Sexualis. With Special Reference to the Antipathic Sexual Instinct: A Medico-Forensic Study.* London: Rebman; 1906.

Wacke A. Fahrlässige Vergehen im römischen Strafrecht. Revue Internationale des Droits de l'Antiquité (RIDA) 1979;26:505−66.

Ziino G. Compendio di medicina legale e giurisprudenza medica secondo le leggi dello Stato ed i più recenti progressi della Scienza ad uso de' medici e giuristi. 3rd ed. Milano: Società editrice libraria; 1890.

CHAPTER 5

Asclepius and the Snake as Toxicological Symbols in Ancient Greece and Rome

Gregory Tsoucalas and George Androutsos

The potential for myth-making has always resided in human consciousness as a means of coping with and explaining the unknown. The mind's capacity for scientific reasoning does not necessarily contradict the need for myth. Mythology constructs a world of logic and illogic, enriched with interconnected stories to conjure up viable personal and social environments [1]. The unlikeliness of a snake with human attributes led to the myth of Asclepius and his companion snake [Figure 5.1]. The snake, by using its venom, could both inflict poisonous wounds and be therapeutic. Asclepius, one of the band of the mythic Greek heroes known as the Argonauts, was expert in all facets of drugs and poisons. Eventually, myth had him evolving into the snake God, and so it was that the snake became the eternal symbol of medicine and toxicology [2].

The 5th century BC in Ancient Greece marked the reappearance of an earlier custom of praising the gods with votive offerings, while palliative measures comprised of magical and divine forces once again became the mainstream approach in medicine. The social changes that ensued at the end of the 5th century BC were favorable for the mythmaking evolution of god-therapists who could help restore health. The individual in need of treatment sought a deity who could heal and cure [3].

Soon, various political and social systems were established to incorporate the individual into the larger community. The people's frustration with the existing deistic framework was especially evident in rural areas of Greece and had its largest impact on the interface of religion and medicine. The Olympian gods with their heroic, brutal, chaotic, and bombastic characteristics were no longer able to meet the needs of the common people, and, as a result, the gods began to take on a less intimidating, softer character [4,5]. During this period, medicine was linked with religion and was under the patronage of one god, Asclepius. The main purpose of the Asclepiadai (Greek: Ασκληπιάδαι)—the physician-priests in

History of Toxicology and Environmental Health. DOI: http://dx.doi.org/10.1016/B978-0-12-801506-3.00005-4

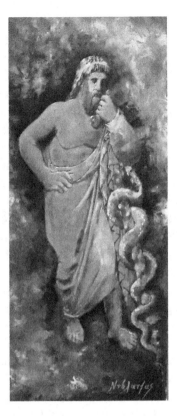

Figure 5.1 Asclepius, a painting by Theodoros Ntolatzas, 2009, Athens, Greece.

the temples of Asclepius—was to renew the human being and keep him healthy. The possibility of divine intervention in dealing with humanity's infirmities was fairly well accepted. Said originally to be a mortal, Asclepius was son of Apollo and a mortal woman, and was ultimately transformed into the primary god for healing. Some say this occurred following his death and resurrection when he became, in a sense, an alter ego of the healing god Apollo [6]. The Ancient Greeks, in worshiping a god who had ascended from their own mortal species, thereby acquired a more personal contact with the divine when it came to dealing with their health problems. This relationship was marked by ceremonies in which votive offerings were combined with a purification bath, herbal fumigation, and sacred temple animals such as the dog, the turtle dove, the rooster, and, above all, the snake [7].

Asclepius is often pictured with a snake-entwined staff [8]. He was undeniably the best known practitioner of medicine in mythology and was said to be able to resurrect the dead, which reflected his strong chthonic nature, reinforced by iconography depicting him with his steadfast companion, the snake [3,9]. Today, about 50 statues depicting Asclepius with his companion are on display in museums around the world [10]. The sacred snake was not simply an emblem for Asclepius. He himself, when he entered the sacred grounds of his temples, would appear transformed into a holy snake, ready to cure the believers [11]. Moreover, the snake was always depicted as the guardian of the temples of the gods, as well as the Oracle of Delphi, where a giant snake, the "Dragon Python," protected the sacred ground [12]. Numerous questions persist: Was the snake ascended from a simple guardian to a healing god? Was the snake Asclepius's alter ego? Was Asclepius himself a famous mythical snake that had once affected a miraculous cure with its venom and then came to be worshiped in human form? Was the snake a poisonous deadly creature, or was the snake a healing demigod? Hypotheses abound, but the answers remain lost forever in the dense fog of Greek mythology. About 200 years later the snake-god, traveling the long mythical route from Epidaurus to Rome, was adopted by the Romans, who called him Aesculapius and made him the symbol of medicine for the entire Roman Empire. Although the Romans worshiped many healing gods, notably Dea Prema, Bona Dea, Carna, and Deus Subigus, Aesculapius was so dominant and revered that he became the first healing god assigned a holy temple on Tiber island [13].

According to Greek myth, Asclepius was the son of Apollo and the nymph Koronis [11,14]. In his youth he became the greatest pupil of the centaur Chiron, the famed teacher of physicians [2,15,16]. On one hand, Apollo was a fearsome god of pestilence; capable of annihilating people by the score; on the other hand, he was a healing god, worshiped by the Greeks in temples where believers, pleading for a cure of their physical ailments, would participate in purification and hypnotization ceremonies [17]. It was the noble Chiron, though, expert in all aspects of medicine, who was the primary tutor of Asclepius [2]. Meanwhile, the goddess Athena gave Asclepius blood from the mythical creature, Medusa, whose head was covered not with hair but with snakes. Athena taught Asclepius how to use the blood from the right vein (snake) as a healing elixir and the blood from the left vein as a deadly poison to "harm people" [18]. It was through this action that the goddess Athena bestowed divine powers on the mortal serpent.

Asclepius thus became the great healer, able to manage the fate of the sick. He could save them or he could condemn them to Hades; he could even bring the dead back to life. Asclepius was almost equal in stature to the Olympian gods and was a famous physician on Mount Pelion, where he had been tutored by Chiron. Soldiers wounded in fierce battles, suffering from serious wounds inflicted by bronze swords or by stones hurled at them, sick people distressed by their suffering, people burned from the summer sun or frozen from the winter cold—all sought relief on Pelion. Asclepius used spells, songs, elixirs, ointments, and drugs, and succeeded in curing them all [19,20]. Knowing that snakes were the guardians of the temples, the gatekeepers that knew everything about the gods, the temples, the priests, and the common people, Asclepius, in his human form, decided to raise a snake of his own. He most probably chose one from Epidaurus, where the snakes were known to be tamer [21], and brought it with him to Pelion to serve as his companion [2]. His life forever after would be closely connected with the snake.

Asclepius, with his ability to resurrect the dead, matching the power of Hades, could transform himself into the holy snake, the guardian that soon became a demigod to be worshiped alongside him in his temples, the Asclepeiia (Greek: Ασκληπιεία) [11]. This transformation suggests that the first form of the new healing god was probably that of a serpent. When summoned by his priests, the Asclepiadai, he would arrive in the form of a giant snake to practice his healing skills. On one occasion the snake-god entered his temple in Epidaurus, where a poor man suffering from a malignant ulcer in his foot, was ready to die. The snake slowly moved toward him and licked the ulcer, while the fluids (i.e., the venom) cured the malignancy [22]. On another occasion, an infertile woman summoned Asclepius for aid. Again in the form of a giant snake he entered the temple, and by cuddling the woman's abdomen he bestowed upon her a fertile future: She would give birth to five strong babies [23].

The fame of the snake-god, Asclepius, reputed to deliver miraculous remedies for almost all ailments, spread throughout Ancient Greece. Votive offerings with spiraling snakes were devoted in large numbers in his name. The poisonous snake-god with his venom could provoke a quick death to express the gods' wrath, or alternatively, he could palliate the sufferer. Asclepiadai reportedly cared for the snakes inside a round peribolos, the abaton (Greek: άβατον: a sanctuary in the center of a temple without a roof) [24]. They also knew how to extract venom from the mouth cavity of the snake and used it in small doses as a therapeutic drug [18,25]. For centuries, the snake had served Apollo and had learned theurgic medicine. For years it was used in the medical training of Asclepius by the Centaur Chiron, an expert both in botany and in the preparation of drugs and poisons. Finally, as previously noted, Athena taught Asclepius how to use Medusa's blood. In his human form, Asclepius practiced the use of drugs to heal and harm. In the end, the snake-god could cure the diseases of the body, spirit, and soul, as well as control the erotic passions. He could hypnotize and treat the sufferers by appearing in their dreams. Asclepius was the founder of a line of physicians, while his alter ego, the snake, became for all time the symbol of healing and toxicology [13].

In 293 BC, after two years of a devastating epidemic in a Roman province, all hopes were on Asclepius. It was his moment of glory to enter the Roman Pantheon, to make his breakthrough to eternity. For two years Lazio (the region of Italy where Rome is located) had suffered horrific deaths among its population, as well as anemia and other diseases. The plethora of the dead, the despair of disease, the suffering of the ill, and the fatigue of the grave diggers drove the Romans to the sanctuary of the Delphic Oracle. The Oracle's prophecy was clear "That which you seek isn't here. You must search for it elsewhere. You don't need Apollo, but in reality you need his son. Go and beg his son." A Roman contingent therefore traveled all the way to Epidaurus where they asked the local lords for aid. While the lords were discussing whether to help them, the snake-god appeared in the dreams of the Romans, advising them: "Don't be afraid, I will abandon my statue and come with you." Subsequently, Asclepius, in the form of a snake, boarded the Roman ship for the long voyage to Rome. Through the River Tiber, he reached the shore near the eternal city, where, as a serpent, he jumped into the water and swam to the island of Tiber. Resuming, at that point, his human form, he cured the sick and saved the people from the pestilence [13,26–28].

The name Asclepius itself reveals a strong connection to snakes. The first part, "Ascl" (Greek: Ασκλ), derives from the word *Ascalavo* (Greek: Ασκάλαβο), which means snake (Greek: όφις or φίδι), while the second part "epius" (Greek: ήπιος) means meek or gentle. The Greek word for snake, όφις (ofis), derives from the Greek word ώφθην (ofthin), which means he who sees everything, the guardian. The sacred snake was also mentioned as a dragon (Greek: δέρκομε, derkome), which means he who possesses excellent vision and understanding, that is. all seeing and all knowing [13]. In Ancient Greek "giras" (Greek: γήρας) means the skin that the snake periodically sheds, but it also means "old age" [29]. Asclepius was an omniscient snake-god, who could see through every disease and could manipulate the healing properties of all drugs; a god who could rejuvenate himself at will by shedding his old skin, the "giras."

It was important for a pharmacist or physician of the era to have deep knowledge of both remedies and poisons. By understanding the snake's own immunity to its deadly venom, many have tried to devise the ultimate potion to treat all kinds of poisoning. King Mithridates the 6th (132−64 BC), in an attempt to protect himself from poisoning, and wanting to strengthen his immune response concocted an antidote consisting of 54 different substances. In an attempt to make himself invulnerable to poisons, he drank small portions of the antidote. This antidote became known as Mithridatiki. It was patterned after the Theriac, an antidote of 64 different substances, prepared in 63 BC, by the pharmacist Krateus, Mithridates' advisor [30−32]. The epic poem by Nicander (197−130 BC), *Theriaca*, includes a chapter titled "Opfiaca" (Greek: Οφιακά, όφις = snake) and deals with the healing potions against snake venom. In time, antidotes aiming to heal all poisons were named "Theriac," the ultimate cure, and many, as Mithridates did, tried to formulate such a cure-all [2].

In Ancient Greece, many figures associated with the underworld were also relevant to fertility. The chthonic goddess Demeter, for example, was also the protector of fertility, while Artemis and Hecate (similar or identical goddesses) were protectors of newborns, and chthonic Apollo was also a god of light (poetic paradox), the healing god of the Ancient Greeks. The snake, apart from crawling on the ground, could enter the earth connecting the mortal world with the underground world of Hades. Its reemergence above ground was the sign of a new birth. The Ancient Greeks were innovative sea pioneers, but they were also an agricultural civilization that strongly valued the earth and the work of sowing and harvesting—a cycle of death and rebirth. For them, the snake encapsulated the most significant values of their culture [33].

In Minoan Crete, the Mother goddess was a symbol of fertility and palliative medicine. She was depicted holding two snakes in her hands, and in some cases she held poppies. The healing powers of the opium poppy were known in Minoan culture and were connected with the snake. The lekythi, a trefoil flask, which had been used to store what was probably liquid opium, usually depicted a snake under its handles [29], suggesting a relationship between opium and snake venom. On the island of Kos, the homeland of Hippocrates, every year the inhabitants celebrated "the rod's ascension," indicating the significance of the physician's walking stick. This wooden shaft was once a weapon for warriors, but later it became not only a supportive instrument, but also a tool symbolizing the physician's readiness to heal, a symbol of life. By adding the snake, a second symbol of life, Asclepius was acknowledged as the primary god of healing, the custodian of health [3,13]. Coins from the Greek island of Cos, which lies on the Aegean Sea a few miles from Crete, often depicted a bearded man holding a walking stick with a snake coiled around it [19,29]. That may have been the origin of the iconography of the physician and the staff-entwined snake. Later, coins from Pergamum and Rome depicting curved snakes, a rod with a snake, or the figure of Asclepius with both of his symbols, appeared with greater frequency [34].

The snake has been recognized as a medical emblem for more than 2500 years. It is featured entwined around a staff of knowledge and wisdom in most images and statues depicting Asclepius [35]. The snake became the symbol of rebirth, the provider of innovative remedies, the bringer of the theriac, and the healing demigod companion of Asclepius (Aesculapius). It was an early example of a binary god who could use venoms and had knowledge of their circulation inside the veins. The snake represented the flow of energy. Being wrapped around the crook of Asclepius, the snake had supported Asclepius in his long voyages. The serpent demigod, who became a binary chthonic god with both serpent and human form, became the insignia of medicine and toxicology for millennia to come. Indeed, it is a totem of life.

REFERENCES

[1] Tsatsos K, Kakridis I, Kiraikidou-Nestoros A. Analysis and interpretation of the Greek Myth. Athens: Ekdotiki Athinon; 1986.

[2] Tsoucalas I. Pediatrics from Homer until Today. Skopelos-Thessaloniki: Science Press; 2004.

[3] Kerényi K. Der göttliche Artz: Studien über Asklepios und seine Kultstätte. Basel: Ciba; 1947.

[4] Bengston H. History of ancient Greece. Athens: Melisa-Gavriilis; 1991.

[5] Boardman J. Suppl. 6 Excavations in Chios 1952–1955. Athens: Greek Emporio; 1967.

[6] Constantelos D. The interface of medicine and religion in the Greek and the Christian Greek Orthodox tradition. Athens: Greek Orthodox Theological Review; 1988.

[7] Aravantinos A. Asclepius and asclepieia. Leipzig: Drougoulinou; 1907.

[8] Papahatzis N. Asclepius the physician. Greek Mythology, The gods. Athens: Ekdotiki Athinon; 1986.

[9] Holtzman B. Asklepios. Munich-Zurich: LIMC II; 1984.

[10] Hamarneh SK. Background of history of Arabic medicine and the allied health science. Yarmouk (Jordan): Yarmouk University; 1986.

[11] Graeciae descriptio. In: Spiro F, editor. Pausaniae Graeciae descriptio, 3 vols. Leipzig: Teubner; 1903 (repr. Stuttgart: 1:1967).

[12] Apollodorus. Bibliotheca 'A. Leipzig: Taubner; 1854.

[13] Pollak K. Die Heilkunde der Antike. Griechenland-Rom-Byzanz. Die Medizin in Bibel und Talmud. Dusseldorf: Econ Verlag; 1969.

[14] Hesiod. Fragmenta. Athens: Pirinos Kosmos; 2007.

[15] Pherecydes. Fragmenta. Leipzig: Altera; 1824.

[16] Philostratus Fl. Olearius. Zurich: Meyer & Zeller; 1844.

[17] Bernheim F, Zener AA. The Sminthian Apollo and the epidemic among the Achaeans at Troy. Trans Am Philol Assoc 1978;108:11−4.

[18] Stagiritis A. Ogygia. (On doctors). John Varth. Vienna: Tsvekiou; 1818.

[19] Krug A. Heilkunst und Heilkult: Medizin in der Aentike. Munich: Beck; 1993.

[20] Doukas N. Comments on Pindar. Athens: Adreou Koromila; 1842.

[21] Tziarou K. Asclepius, The god of medicine. Medical Podium J 2006;3:94−101.

[22] Epigraph IG IV(2),1 [Epidauros] 121 115−118.

[23] Epigraph IG IV(2),1 [Epidauros] 122 117−119.

[24] Campbell J. Spirit and nature. London: Routledge and Kegan Paul; 1955.

[25] Angeletti LR. Views of classical medicine. Theurgical and secular rational medicine in the healing-temples of ancient Greece. Forum Genova 1991;2:1−11.

[26] Ovidius P. Metamorphosis. Boston: Cornhill Publishing Co; 1922.

[27] Brouwer HJ. Bona Dea. Leiden: E. J. Brill; 1989.

[28] Fairbanks A. The mythology of Greece and Rome. New York: Appleton; 1907.

[29] Ramoutsaki I, Haniotakis S, Tsatsakis A. The snake as the symbol of medicine, toxicology and toxinology. Vet Human Toxicol 2000;42(5):306−8.

[30] Vasileiou RP, Papavasileiou IT. Handbook of the history of medicine. Athens: Athens University Press; 1979.

[31] Gottlob KK. Galen, Opera omnia. Leipzig: Cnoblochii; 1827.

[32] Karaberopoulos D, Karamanou M, Androutsos G. The theriac in antiquity. Lancet 2012;379:1942−3.

[33] Rethimiotakis G. Minon shrine. Archaeol J 1997;134:177 Athens.

[34] Hart GD. Asclepius, god of medicine. Can Med Assoc J 1965;92:232−6.

[35] Antoniou SA, Antoniou GA, Learney R, Granderath FA, Antoniou AI. The rod and the serpent: history's ultimate healing symbol. World J Surg 2011;35:217−21.

CHAPTER 6

Drugs, Suppositories, and Cult Worship in Antiquity

David Hillman

6.1 INTRODUCTION

The oldest Greco-Roman medicines were plant-derived chemicals and animal toxins used predominantly in gynecology and obstetrics.[1] Female physicians, priestesses, and midwives belonged to the oldest pre-Hippocratic traditions of medicine and pharmacy in the Mediterranean and were largely responsible for the establishment of western medicine and pharmacy.

Scholars have closely examined drugs used as potables, edibles, and inhalations, but little is known of the vaginal and anal suppositories used in antiquity, their unique methods of administration, or their use in cultic sexual practices. Despite the under-researched nature of these drugs—due in large part to their direct association with practices and bodily functions considered taboo by modern cultures—a knowledge of their use helps to paint a more complete picture of the historical nexus of drugs and ancient cults as well as the gynecological sophistication of classical civilization.

6.2 DRUGS AND CULTS

Virgil's *Aeneid* preserves a mythic episode that aptly illustrates the predominant role of exotic botanicals and venoms in antiquity as well as

---

[1] Our earliest Greek medical sources include treatises on the proper regulation of menstruation, conception, and delivery. The Hippocratic *Nature of Women* (Περὶ Γυναικείησ Φύσιος) contains lengthy instructions on the preparation and application of pessaries, douches, and other gynecological drugs. The names of gynecological drugs are among the most prominent within the corpus of Greco-Roman pharmacy. Some botanical components of these widely used drugs and drug concoctions derived their common names from the gynecological activity they promoted: for example, the plant known as "aristolochia" means "best childbirth." The nexus of drugs, gynecology, and religion dates back to the foundation of Greco-Roman culture. See Ref. [1]. Greek and Roman myth and cult rites actively promote the use of gynecological drugs in association with the worship of the earliest Mediterranean deities, including mother goddesses, witches, and oracles [8].

History of Toxicology and Environmental Health. DOI: http://dx.doi.org/10.1016/B978-0-12-801506-3.00006-6

their connection with traditional cults. Ancient mystery rites referenced in numerous Greek and Roman poets illustrate the use of potent drugs that affect human sexuality; many of these drugs were applied to the anus and vagina by means of medicated dildos and as pessaries.

Virgil's treatment of the goddess Allecto illustrates the use of drugs within the context of ancient cult ritual. Allecto, a Fury, was very much the quintessential sibyl.[2] Like the goddess Justice, she was an eternally youthful dancer, possessed of the bloom of life, whose mind was immovably set on the "purgation" of the unjust; as an avenging Fury, she sang of the beauty of pain—a psychic pain she imposed as punishment upon the impious.

Virgil described Allecto as one of the daughters of Black Night; she was a Fury who exercised a power to overthrow the sanity of mortals irredeemably possessed by greed, ill-will, and hubris. When heaven needed brother to fight brother, it summoned Allecto; in the seventh book of the *Aeneid*, Juno called upon the teenage goddess to drive a queen crazy in order to start an uncivil war between the inhabitants of Italy and the Trojans.[3]

Allecto spread her maddening poison by applying a snake-derived drug to a mortal woman's biological "pocket," or in Virgil's words, the location of her most intimate sensations. Like other Bacchants, the goddess removed the venom from her own hair, which was traditionally depicted in both art and literature as being full of vipers.[4] After this venom was absorbed vaginally, Virgil says it coursed through the queen's body, intoxicated her, and sent her into an ecstatic frenzy.

---

[2]The figure of Allecto as the virgo or κόρη is foreshadowed in the Etruscan maiden figure of Vanth, who is a combination of Hecate and the Furies. See *The Religion of the Etruscans*, ed. by Grummond and Simon [6]. There is also an element of the Lasas in Allecto, who are known to carry the alabastron (ἀλάβαστρον), an overtly sexual device used to apply μύρον as seen in Aristophanes' *Lysistrata*. The alabastron was mentioned in the gospel of Mark as a perfume container possessed by Mary Magdalene, an alleged prostitute.

[3]Virgil, *Aeneid*, 7.341-7: "Then Allecto, saturated with the poisons of the Gorgons ... takes up a position at the most private portal of queen Amata ... into whom the goddess forcefully inserts a single measure of snake venom taken from her black hair; she applies the suppository in her body's natural pocket, at the place of her most intimate being." Author's translation.

[4]As seen in Aeschylus' *Eumenides* and Euripides' *Bacchae*. Interestingly, most of the deities associated with ritual Bacchic worship were young girls who had not yet had children, yet each was able—like the Nymphs—to provide breast milk to their charges. These nurses are directly associated with the viper of Dionysus, and it is known that viper venom produces a prolactin-like response in mammary tissue.

6.3 BACCHANTS AND VIPER VENOM

Before ancient seers summoned spirits like Allecto from the underworld—an arcane practice known as necromancy—they invoked Bacchus, the god of ecstatic dance. The worship of this mystery cult divinity, known variously as Dionysus, Bromius, and Zagreus, was connected in classical literature and art with the handling of the European horned viper (*Vipera ammodytes*). This snake accompanied Maenads and Bacchants in their religious processions and was frequently associated with young, virgin girls of myth who nursed gods and heroes alike.

In antiquity, snakes like the horned viper were closely bound up with the practice of medicine and the exercises of cults. The Greeks, Romans, and Etruscans did not openly distinguish between the practice of medicine and religion, and even the goddess of health herself—Hygeia—was sometimes portrayed with a snake positioned over an offering dish in a posture that appears to imply the act of milking the animal's venom.

The use of viper venom in ancient medicine and cults may explain how young girls associated with the cult of Bacchus, who were not previously pregnant, were able to function as wet nurses. Crotoxin is a phospholipase A2 neurotoxin produced by a South American pit viper (*Crotalus durissus terrificus*). This crotalid toxin has similar biological activities to the components of horned viper venom and acts on mammary epithelial cells to stimulate the secretion of casein using the same biochemical pathways as prolactin.[5] Stimulating the production of breast milk by the application of viper venom may have been responsible for the ability of these nonparturient girls to lactate.

Divinities like the Furies—one of whom was Allecto—and their sisters, the Death-Spirits (Keres), were represented as being infused with viper venom; the ancient world believed these female entities were particularly hearty and possessed significant stamina, longevity, and an apparent immunity to weakness or illness. Some of them are even called "dragonesses," and are involved with the "burning off" of human mortality. It appears that the priestesses of Hecate, Priapus, and Demeter/Persephone were involved in the consumption of viper

---

[5]See Ref. [2].

venom.[6] These priestesses were considered to be physically superior to ordinary mortals, and like the Furies were of a superior physical constitution—and somewhat immune to disease. Interestingly, crotoxin has shown itself to be a potential anticancer drug.[7]

6.4 ANCIENT VAGINAL SUPPOSITORIES

Allecto's application of a snake-venom-based drug to a woman's vagina is in direct step with ancient gynecological practices. According to the author of the Hippocratic treatise titled *The Nature of Women*, numerous compound drug mixtures in antiquity were used to produce abortion, control uterine bleeding, and treat disease. These drugs were applied directly to the vagina by means of cylindrical pessaries.[8]

Frankincense, myrrh, and blister beetle were all common ingredients in gynecological drug mixtures. Aromatic botanicals were exceptionally common as basic components of Greco-Roman suppositories, unguents, and ointments.

Blister beetle was a very popular aphrodisiac in antiquity just as it has been in the modern world. Cantharidin, a terpenoid secreted by blister beetles, is an irritant or blistering agent that induces priapism. Cantharidin can cause gastrointestinal and renal dysfunction, but it has been used since classical antiquity as an effective aphrodisiac.[9]

Rose oil, like other fragrant volatile oils, was most often used as a base for gynecological applications. The combination of a drug like cantharidin with aromatic oils may have been responsible for the abortifacient and/or contraceptive qualities of these aphrodisiacs. The caustic properties of cantharidin would have irritated the lining of the uterus to such a degree as to induce sloughing and therefore the prevention of implantation. Rose oil concoctions were typically associated

---

[6]*Aeschylus was nearly executed for revealing the secrets of the Eleusinian mysteries in his plays on Orestes. One of these plays (The Cup-bearers) contains a dream of a "dragoness" in which her breast milk is injected with the venom of a snake.*

[7]See Ref. [3].

[8]Hippocrates, *Nature of Women*, 71: "Irritating suppositories that draw blood: mix frankincense and myrrh with blister beetle, forming them as a big as an oak gall; make into an elongated shape, attach it around a feather with a flock of wool, tie it with a thread of fine linen, soak in white Egyptian unguent or rose unguent, and apply." Translated by Paul Potter [8].

[9]Cantharidin has also been used in China. For its history and toxicology see Ref. [4].

with the priestly followers of Aphrodite, who were typically associated with temple prostitution.

According to the aforementioned passage from the Hippocratic *The Nature of Women*, vaginal suppositories were compounded and then worked into a penis-like shape for the sake of application. These drugs were used to affect reproductive physiology, sexual activity, and disease. Greek and Latin vocabulary concerned with suppository usage was highly specific. For example, both cultures employed specific verbs denoting the act of applying of suppositories to the vagina and anus.[10]

6.5 DRUGS AND SEXUALITY

Dioscorides, a first century CE physician and compounder of botanical and animal-derived drugs, wrote at length about the use of oils, ointments, and unguents in sexual contexts. These drugs were typically divided into compounds that "harden" and "soften" the external genitalia—also known as "heating" and "cooling" drugs. The Greco-Roman world used these substances to prepare the genitalia for copulation, to prevent disease and to regulate menstruation; these drugs, despite their numerous varied uses, were known collectively as "aphrodisiacs."

Opobalsamum, known to biblical scholars as the "balm of Gilead," was one such valuable aphrodisiac. According to Dioscorides, opobalsamum was the hard-to-collect exudate of a Middle Eastern tree—a substance produced in response to structural injury.[11] Like the "tears" of myrrh, frankincense, and even the opium poppy, this drug was a potent secondary metabolite that was harvested, packaged, and sold in markets throughout the Mediterranean.[12] Dioscorides reveals that expensive drugs like opobalsamum were so valuable that they were frequently adulterated by drug sellers.[13]

---

[10]"Προστίθημι" in Greek and "subdo" in Latin denote the application of a pessary or a suppository. The Greek gynecological texts found in the Hippocratic corpus—which could not have been written by Hippocratic physicians due to their liberal use of abortifacients—are full of the nominal forms of this verb and associated nouns that indicate or denote a "pessary" or "suppository" [8].

[11]Dioscorides, *De Materia Medica*, 1.19 [7].

[12]Many of the exudates harvested from injury are referred to as "tears" due to their appearance and the fact that they drip slowly from incisions made in the botanicals whence they are derived.

[13]According to Dioscorides, opobalsamum was so valuable that it was worth twice its weight in silver. 1.19. Because of this, he speaks extensively about the best means of testing the drug in order to determine its purity [7].

Opobalsamum—among other things—was a diuretic, an abortifa-cient, and used to treat abrasions of the vulva.[14] Like other secondary metabolites, opobalsamum possessed distinct antifungal and bacterio-static properties that may have been responsible for its use as a means of decreasing the prevalence of certain sexually transmitted diseases. It is also significant that an ointment compounded of opobalsamum was also believed to counteract snake venom—something to which ancient priestesses, like those who worshipped Bacchus, Hecate, and Allecto, would have been exposed.

6.6 APHRODISIAC SUPPOSITORIES AND MAGIC

Priestesses who served divinities like the infernal Furies, or their leader, the witch goddess Hecate, were known in antiquity to exercise powers over demons; such manipulation of the natural world was considered to be the practice of magic. Just as ancient magic was not distinguished from the practice of religion, the use of drugs and the act of sex were not considered to be strictly secular or nonreligious operations; sex, drugs, and religion were a single entity in the ancient world.

According to Petronius, the first century CE author of the *Satyricon*, Roman priestesses were known for their drug-induced sex-ual practices. In one particular episode of his novel, Petronius allows one of his characters to illustrate the power of the priestess-sorceress to control and manipulate human sexuality by means of drugs:

> *"Oenoethea, drawing out a leathern prick, dipped it in a medley of oil, small pepper, and the bruised seed of nettles, and proceeded by degrees to direct its passage through my hinder parts.... with this mixture the old woman labori-ously sprinkled my thighs; ...and with the juice of cresses and southern-wood washing my loins, she took a bunch of green nettles and began to strike gently all the vale below my navel.[15]*

In actuality, the sorceress Oenoethea was acting as a priestess-physician in this passage; she was attempting to cure Petronius' charac-ter of his impotency. What is most curious about the passage is that Petronius does not seem to question the reality that men were readily penetrated anally in medico-religious acts in antiquity. In other words,

---

[14]Dioscorides, *De Materia Medica*, 1.19 [7].
[15]Petronius, *Satyricon*, 138. Translated by W.H.D. Rouse [10].

it was acceptable for men to have drugs applied anally by means of medicated dildos.

The use of nettles both externally and internally as a promoter of penile erection may be the result of the presence of 3,4-Divanillyltetrahydrofuran, a lignan that appears to liberate available testosterone and thus may influence sexual drive.[16]

Medico-religious ceremonies also employed the use of drugs with the intent of producing magical "fluids." Bodily secretions like semen, vaginal ejaculate, saliva, and even breast milk were all important ingredients of magical ceremonies—including healing acts, exorcisms, and "purgations."[17] In another episode found in the *Satyricon*, Petronius causes his characters to employ magic in order to induce erection and ejaculation:

> Then the old woman took a twist of threads of different colors out of her dress, and tied it around my neck. Then she mixed some dust with spittle, and took it on her middle finger, and made a mark on my forehead despite my protest.... after this chant she ordered me to spit three times and throw stones into my bosom three times, after she had said a spell over them and wrapped them in purple and laid her hands on me and proceeded to try the force of their charm on the powers of my groin. Before you could say a word, my sinews obeyed her comment and filled the old woman's hands with a huge upstir.[18]

Like the Fury Allecto, the sorceress in this passage employs magical elements including drugs, incantations, the manipulation of the sexual organs, and the use of body fluids to affect a change in her subject. And once again, the manipulation of sexuality by means of drugs and ritual magic is forced. In other words, Virgil's Allecto inspires madness by means of violently forceful sexual drug-magic, just as Petronius' sorceresses aggressively apply medicines in order to manipulate sexual experience in a religious setting.

6.7 CONCLUSION

The ultimate purpose of using drugs and magical ritual to affect human sexual experience was the veneration of deities. Greek and

---

[16]For a closer look at lignans, see Ref. [5].
[17]The roots of these practices are found in Egypt. See *The Mechanics of Ancient Egyptian Magical Practice* by Robert Ritner [9].
[18]Petronius, *Satyricon*, 131. Translated by W.H.D. Rouse [10].

Roman sorceresses worked with one goal in mind; they desired to celebrate the gods by using magic to create oracular vision. Vaginal suppositories that maddened women, anally inserted medicated dildos that mesmerized men, and drugs used to force the expulsion of ejaculate were all elements of the creation of religious song.

Religious ecstasy was enhanced by drugs and the rituals of young priestesses, but the climactic moment of ancient medico-religious experience was always accompanied by a divine utterance or shout. This shout became the holy voice of the deity overseeing the performance of such mysteries; the god was directly served by means of this ecstatic vocalization. In other words, when Allecto forcefully drugged her victims by penetrating their most private body parts, and thus infused them with fury, their pained screams of lunatic agony served Justice.

REFERENCES

[1] Riddle J. Goddesses, elixirs, and witches: plants and sexuality throughout human history. New York, NY: Palgrave Macmillan; 2010.

[2] Ollivier-Bousquet M, Radvanyi F, Bon C. Crotoxin, a phospholipase A2 neurotoxin from snake venom, interacts with epithelial mammary cells, is internalized and induces secretion. Mol Cell Endocrinol 1991;82(1):41−50.

[3] Jorge E. Cura, Daniel P. Blanzaco, Cecilia Brisson. Phase I and pharmacokinetics study of crotoxin (cytotoxic PLA2, NSC-624244) in patients with advanced cancer1. Clin Cancer Res 2002;8:1033.

[4] Moed L, Shwayder TA, Chang MW. Cantharidin revisited: a blistering defense of an ancient medicine. Arch Dermatol 2001;137.

[5] Touré A, Xueming X. Flaxseed lignans: source, biosynthesis, metabolism, antioxidant activity, bio-active components, and health benefits. Compr Rev Food Sci Food Saf 2010;9 (3):261−9.

[6] De Grummond N, Simon E, editors. The religion of the Etruscans. Austin, TX: University of Texas Press; 2006.

[7] Dioscorides P. De materia medica. Berlin: August Raabe; 1958.

[8] Potter P, editor. Hippocrates, vol. X. Cambridge: Harvard University Press; 2012.

[9] Ritner RK. The mechanics of ancient Egyptian magical practice. Chicago, IL: University of Chicago; 1993, Studies in Ancient Oriental Civilization, No. 54.

[10] Warmington EH, editor. Petronius: Satyricon; Seneca: Apocolocyntosis [Rouse WHD, Trans.]. Cambridge: Harvard University Press; 1987.

CHAPTER 7

Kohl Use in Antiquity: Effects on the Eye

Zafar Alam Mahmood, Iqbal Azhar and S. Waseemuddin Ahmed

7.1 INTRODUCTION

Exploring the history of ancient civilizations is still relevant today, helping us learn valuable lessons regarding both their achievements and their failures. Some of the oldest civilizations had a surprisingly sophisticated knowledge of science, but how they reached such a level of understanding remains a mystery. The history of ophthalmology and ophthalmic products provides one example of diverse classical preparations still used in alternative systems of medicines in different parts of the world. The use of kohl throughout history illustrates that many ancient civilizations had sound knowledge of science. Over the centuries, kohl was used under different names and both men and women of all socioeconomic levels made use of it.

Comprehensive details relating to the eye and its diseases, including eye treatments in ancient Egypt, have been amply documented in various scientific reviews, highlighting the application and role of lead-based eye preparations, kohl [1,2]. However, no specific reviews or research articles have yet been published authenticating lead poisoning in ancient Egypt or in any other ancient civilization. If we assume that use of kohl was pervasive in ancient Egypt, can we conclude that everyone in Egypt was a victim of lead poisoning? Certainly not. Scientists still need more data to explore the benefits and toxicity of kohl. The questions most people ask today relate to its constituents, dating, mechanism, and effect; that is, what kind of materials were used to manufacture kohl, when and where was it made, how does it work and what effects does its application produce in the eyes.

The exact composition of kohl has long been an important topic and a matter of dispute within the scientific community. German and French scientists have played a prominent role in authenticating the exact chemical nature of kohl through chemical analysis, electron

History of Toxicology and Environmental Health. DOI: http://dx.doi.org/10.1016/B978-0-12-801506-3.00007-8

microscopy, and X-ray diffraction [2–6]. During Egyptian rule, galena was known by the name *mestem* or *stim*; the latter word is identical to the Greek, *stimmi* or *stibi*, and to the Latin *stibium*, meaning antimony [3]. Therefore, some authors have misinterpreted or, rather, mixed these words and reported antimony as the active ingredient, instead of lead sulfide. The controversy regarding the chemical composition of kohl was finally resolved after the publication of Professor V. X. Fischer's research article [3] in which he analyzed 30 samples of ancient Egyptian eye preparations (kohls) obtained from Fayum (Egypt) and demonstrated that galena was indeed the chief constituent. In view of this clear evidence, there can be no doubt that the word *stibium* referred primarily to galena (lead sulphide) and not to antimony [7,8]. Another analytical report, this one by French scientists [4], confirmed the presence of galena and other lead salts after analyzing a huge number of samples (dating from between 2000 and 1200 BC) that were preserved in their original containers. The crystallographic and chemical analysis indicated the presence of galena (PbS), along with some quantity of cerussite ($PbCO_3$) and two synthetic products, laurionite (PbOHCl) and phosgenite ($Pb_2Cl_2CO_3$), reflecting the Egyptians' extensive knowledge of "wet" chemistry.

Galena is found near the Red Sea, Aswan, and the Eastern Desert at Gebel-el-Zeit, and Gebel Rasas, also known as Lead Mountain [9]. Figure 7.1 pictures the Egyptian, Sinai, and Arab Peninsula and Galena's possible trade route into Egypt (North Africa) and the Middle East [10]. No evidence of antimony mines was found in Egypt, Sinai, Saudi Arabia, or Iran. Instead, antimony mines have been identified in Macedonia, Turkey, and Armenia. Apparently, the galena used to prepare kohl in both the Egyptian and the Arabian Peninsula was brought from the two large mines located in Egypt. There is little chance that antimony brought from Macedonia, Turkey, or Armenia was used by the Egyptians and Arabs to manufacture kohl. This further supports the earlier statement that antimony was mistaken for galena and that galena was the actual ingredient of kohl, which its manufacturers still use today.

Studies of the medicinal properties of natural substances used during medieval and Ottoman times also show that galena was used to cure eye diseases [11]. Evidence relating to the composition of kohl is cited in *The Encyclopaedia of Islam* [12] and in *Medieval Islamic Civilization—An Encyclopaedia* [13]. The various literatures of the time

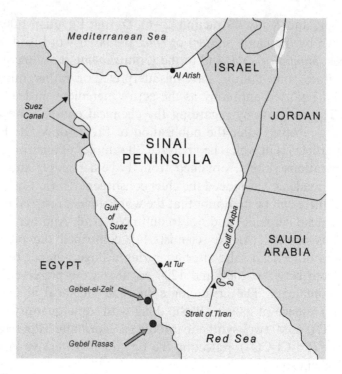

Figure 7.1 Showing location of Jabel Rasas and Gebel-el-Zeit on the Red sea coast.

report differing opinions as to the relative benefits and toxicity of kohl. The scientific community posits that an intellectual war arose between two schools of thoughts. The first proposed that since lead is toxic, it was likely hazardous for the human body and should not be used even in eye preparations, regardless of the type of lead (organic or inorganic), and its physicochemical behavior and route of application. The second school of thought maintained that lead toxicity relates to organic lead (such as tetraethyl lead or tetramethyl lead) or some soluble inorganic lead salts. Moreover, it was believed that the inorganic lead in galena was an insoluble lead salt; it had been used for thousands of years owing to its biomedical importance and was not toxic when applied to the eyes in the form of kohl because of its physicochemical nature and mode of action. The first school of thought based its premises primarily on the detection of lead sulfide in various kohl preparations collected from different geographical regions. As additional support for their perspective, members of this school stated that if kohl were misused, there could be an indirect relationship between its application and lead toxicity. Thus, although some studies on children have concluded that kohl may produce toxicity, they have not been controlled studies, nor have they taken into account the environmental, nutritional, and other relevant factors of the region and people.

In contrast, the second school of thought contends that there is a scientific basis for the application of kohl, a centuries-old preparation, and that it certainly has biomedical importance when applied to the eyes. In support of this belief, a number of controlled research trials conducted on both humans and animals have been published suggesting that kohl applied in the eyes does not increase blood lead levels, nor do the studies show that kohl produces any toxicity. There are some reports [14] of minute conjunctival abrasion when lead sulphide (galena) is applied in the form of an eye preparation (kohl/surma), possibly due to substandard products having larger particle size, but no toxic injury. An extensive literature search done to investigate the issue of kohl's toxicity has been reported in a review article [8]. It should be noted that, as a protective agent, the lead in kohl promotes the production of nitric oxide (diatomic free radicle), which is known to boost the immune system's response to infection.

Kohl has been closely associated with almost all human civilizations. Its use dates back to the Bronze Age (3500-1100 BC), and it is even mentioned in the Old Testament (see Kings II 9:30 and Ezekiel 23:40, particularly the reference to "painted eyes"). The word "kohl" is Arabic in origin; Arab oculists called it Kahal [15]. It was accepted by people of many ancient civilizations, including the Sumerians (3500-1950 BC in Iraq), Egyptians (3050-30 BC), Greeks (1550-100 BC), Romans (753 BC-AD 476), Chinese (2100 BC-1911 AD), Japanese (1800-1500 BC), Phoenicians (1200-146 BC in Lebanon), Persians (569-330 BC), Indians (1500 BC), and Muslims (AD 641). Its use continued right through to the Coptic Period (the phase of Christian Egyptian culture) which lasted from the end of the Roman Period (the end of the 3rd century AD) to the coming of Islam AD 641. Kohl is indeed one of the most ancient ophthalmological preparations known to humans.

The effects of kohl on the eyes have been reviewed by many research workers during the last 50 years. The classical views of two schools of thoughts have been described above. For a more detailed explanation, we have examined two of the most important effects of kohl: the protective effect of kohl against UV radiation from the sun and its antimicrobial action for both therapeutic and prophylactic purposes.

7.2 PROTECTIVE EFFECT AGAINST UV RADIATION

The UV absorptive property of galena in the deserts of the Sinai-Egyptian and Arabian Peninsula has been highlighted by many researchers. Galena's black, shiny particles have been reported to screen the eyes from the brilliance and reflection of sunlight and thus protect the eyes from the harmful effect of the sun's UV rays and the flies in the deserts [16–19]. A series of reviews and studies also document galena's solar absorption properties [20,21], thus supporting the ancient civilization's application of kohl to protect their eyes from sun, especially in the deserts of the Sinai-Egyptian and Arab Peninsula. Scientific evidence regarding the absorption and transmittance rate of sunrays by lead sulphide is available and can be used to correlate the solar protective property of kohl when applied to the eyes [20,21]. The light absorption spectrum of a thin film of lead sulfide prepared on indium tin oxide (ITO) is reported to be high and low in transmittance in the UV band, which further increases with deposition voltage [22]. This implies that lead sulfide's thin film will have higher absorption and lower transmittance in the UV light band. Therefore, when kohl (which is made up of lead sulfide) is applied to the eyes as a thin film, it should react similarly, thus absorbing the sun's UV light and protecting the eyes from its harmful effects.

Lead sulfide has been reported to be an important direct narrow-gap semiconductor material with an energy band gap of $-0.4\,eV$ at 300 K and a relatively large excitation Bohr radius of 18 nm. These properties also make lead sulfide suitable for infrared (IR) detection applications [23]. These findings offer reasonable justification to conclude that kohl containing lead sulfide as a major ingredient has a natural protective effect against the sun's glare when applied to the eyes in the form of kohl and thus support claims and uses reported elsewhere. The role of other ingredients of kohl was also investigated. Some interesting formulations reflecting the benefits of these ingredients for the eyes are reported elsewhere in the literature. For example, zinc oxide was probably used in kohl because of its powerful natural sun-block property [24], and it may enhance the protective capacity of galena against the glare of the sun. Interestingly, zinc oxide is a modern sunscreen ingredient. Neem (*Azadirachta indica*) is very well known worldwide for its astringent and antibacterial properties [25,26]. Like silver leaf, neem also possesses antiviral activity [27].

7.3 ANTIMICROBIAL ACTION AND BIOMEDICAL IMPORTANCE

Although the antimicrobial action of kohl was known for centuries, inasmuch as the Egyptians used it to protect against eye infection, recently a more scientific approach has been launched to establish kohl's antimicrobial action. French researchers have reported that the heavy kohl-based eye makeup that the ancient Egyptians used for centuries may actually have had some medical benefits. At low dose, the specially made lead compounds actually boost the immune system by stimulating production of nitric oxide [2]. During the last 30 years, nitric oxide has been recognized as an extremely versatile agent in the immune system [28]. At the time of its discovery (1985–1990), nitric oxide was simply defined as a product of macrophage activated by cytokines. With the passage of time, however, its role has now been broadened to include antimicrobial [29–31], anti-tumor [32–36], and anti-inflammatory–immunosuppressive activity [28,33,37–44]. Nitric oxide is reported to possess broad-spectrum antibacterial activity. This property is based primarily on two reactive by-products, peroxynitrite ($ONOO^-$) and dinitrogen trioxide (N_2O_3). Nitric oxide is quite effective on both Gram-positive and Gram-negative bacteria, including methicillin-resistant *Staphylococcus aureus* [29]. It is now well established that nitric oxide (NO) is an endogenous cell-signaling molecule of fundamental importance in physiology, and so it has become the subject of considerable scientific interest in recent years. There is evidence that certain diseases are related to a deficiency in the production of nitric oxide. This creates the possibility of developing new drug treatments that can donate nitric oxide when the body cannot generate sufficient amounts to permit normal biological functions. NO and other molecules involved in NO-mediated signaling are present in ocular tissues. Studies have shown that topical or systemic administration of classic NO-donors (nitroglycerine, isosorbide dinitrate) in patients reduce intraocular pressure (IOP), supporting a role for nitric oxide in regulating IOP [45–48]. This finding is of particular interest in the potential treatment of glaucoma, which is often associated with an increased IOP and can lead to blindness if not treated.

The antimicrobial activity of nitric oxide has been shown to take place through several mechanism. This activity may be the result of

DNA mutation; inhibition of DNA repair and synthesis or inhibition of protein synthesis; alteration of proteins by S-nitrosylation; ADP-ribosylation or tyrosine nitration or inactivation of enzymes by disruption of Fe-S clusters, zinc fingers, or heme groups; or by peroxidation of membrane lipids [28]. Unfortunately, nitric oxide cannot as yet be used as a drug due to its very short half- life (only a couple of seconds). However, scientists are working on delivering this chemical through nanotechnology. Nitric oxide is soluble in both aqueous and lipid media and thus readily diffuses through the cytoplasm and plasma membranes. Figure 7.2 is based on studies by French scientists and others, and reports on heavy metal ions, such as Pb2 + as well as the release of nitric oxide and its effect on eyes. Amazingly, many scientists now believe that the ancient Egyptians were aware of the beneficial effects of galena-based kohl.

After the publication of the paper by the French scientists, Tapsoba and colleagues [2], a number of web-based reviews and one review article published opposing opinions. It is of course very difficult to unequivocally demonstrate that the ancient Egyptians were familiar with the role of NO, when kohl is applied to the eyes therapeutically, but several papers [1,4−8] have indicated that the Egyptians were quite aware of various diseases and their treatment. Even today, some pharmaceutical companies manufacture ophthalmic products based on nitric oxide activity.

According to ancient Egyptian manuscripts, lead-based eye preparations were essential remedies for treating eye illness. This conclusion seems astonishing to us today when we consider the well-recognized toxicity of lead salts. French scientists, using microelectrodes, obtained new insight into the biochemical interactions between lead (II) ions and cells, which support the ancient medical use of insoluble or sparingly soluble lead compounds. In Tapsoba's study [2], it was reported that a submicromolar concentration of Pb2 + ions is sufficient to elicit a specific oxidative stress response of keratinocytes, leading to overproduction of NO. Based on NO's established biological role in stimulating nonspecific immunological defenses, it can be concluded that lead-based eye preparations (kohl) were manufactured and used in ancient Egypt to prevent and treat eye illnesses by supporting the immune system [2].

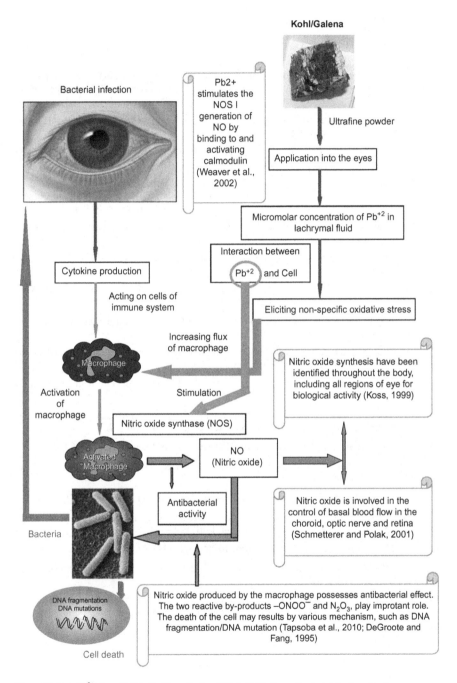

Figure 7.2 Role Pb²⁺ from Kohl in the biosynthesis of Nitric Oxide for antibacterial & other effects.

REFERENCES

[1] Anderson SR. History of Ophthalmology, The eye and its diseases in ancient Egypt. Acta Ophthalmol Scand 1997;75:338−44.

[2] Tapsoba I, Arbault S, Walter P, Amatore C. Finding out Egyptian God's secret using analytical chemistry: biomedical properties of Egyptian black makeup relealed by amperometry at single cells. Anal Chem 2010;82:457−60.

[3] Fischer VX. The chemical composition of ancient Egyptian eye preparations (English Translation). Arch Pharm 1892;230:9−38.

[4] Walter P, Martinetto P, Tsoucaris G, Brniaux R, Lefebvre MA, Richard G, et al. Making make-up in ancient Egypt. Nature 1999;397:483−4.

[5] Martinetto P, Anne M, Dooryhee E, Tsoucaris G, Walter P. A synchrotron X-ray diffraction study of Egyptian cosmetics. In: Creagh DC, Bradley DA, editors. Radiation in Art and Archeometry. Amsterdam, The Netherlands: Published by Elsevier; 2000. p. 297−316.

[6] Habibullah P, Mahmood ZA, Sualeh M, Zoha SMS. Studies on the chemical composition of kohl stone by X-ray defractometer. Pak J PharmSci 2010;23(1):48−52.

[7] Lucas A, Harris J. Ancient Egyptian materials and industries. Courier Dover Publications; 2012.

[8] Mahmood ZA, Zoha SMS, Usmanghani K, Hasan MM, Ali O, Jhan S, et al. Kohl (Surma): retrospect and prospect. Pak J Pharm Sci 2009;22(1):107−22.

[9] Pauline WT. Ancient Egyptian costume history, Part 6- Ancient Egyptian make up and cosmetics, <www.fashion-era.com>; 2007.

[10] Catherine CJ. Kohl as traditional women's adornment in North Africa and Middle East, Introduction to Harquus: Part 2: Kohl. 2005. p.1−9.

[11] Lev E. Reconstructed material medica of the Medieval and Ottoman Al-sham. J Ethnopharmacol 2002;80:167−79.

[12] Bosworth CE, Donzel EV, Lewis B, Pellat C. The Encyclopedia of Islam. Prepared under the patronage of the International Union of Academics. 1986;5:356−57.

[13] Meri JW. Cosmetic. In: Medieval Islamic Civilization − An Encyclopedia. 2006;1:177.

[14] Grant WM, Schuman JS. Toxicology of the eye. 4th ed. Springfield, Illinois: Charles C Thomas; 1993. p. 682−685.

[15] Sweha F. Kohl along history in medicine and cosmetics. Hist Sci Med 1982;17(2):182−3.

[16] Heather CR. Art of arabian costume − a saudi arabian profile. Information on Kohl application. Saudi Arabia: Arabesque Commercial; 1981. p. 1−188.

[17] Cohen M. Cosmetics and perfumes, Egypt. 10,000 BCE 1999.

[18] Kathy C. An A to Z of places and things Saudi. Published by Stacey International Stacey International; 2001. p. 139.

[19] Cartwright-Jones C. Introduction to Harquus: Part 2: Kohl as traditional women's adornment in North Africa and the Middle East. Ohio: TapDancing Lizard Publications; 2005.

[20] Nir A, Tamir A, Zelnik N, Iancu TC. Is eye cosmetic a source of lead poisoning? Isr J Med Sci 1992;28(7):417−21.

[21] Pop I, Nascu C, Lonescu V. Structural and optical properties of PbS thin films obtained by chemical deposition. Thin Solid Films 1997;307:240−4.

[22] Li-Yun C, Wen H, Jian-Feng H, Jian-Peng W. Influence of deposition voltage on properties of lead sulfide thin film. Am Ceram Soc Bull 2008;87(6):9101−4.

[23] Gadenne P, Yagil Y, Deutscher G. Transmittance and reflection in-situ measurements of semicontinuous gold film during deposition. J Appl Phys 1989;66:3019.

[24] Mitchnick MA, Fairhurst D, Pinnell SR. Microfine zinc oxide (Z-Cote) as a photostable UVA/UVB sunblock agent. J Am Acad Dermatol 1999;40:85−90.

[25] Almas K. The antimicrobial effects of extract of *Azadirachta indica* (neem) and *Salvadora persica* (arak) chewing sticks. Indian J Dent Res 1999;10(1):23−6.

[26] Linda SR. Mosby's handbook of herbs & natural supplements. Mosbey; 2001. p. 616−618.

[27] Badam L, Joshi SP, Bedekar SS. In vitro antiviral activity of neem (Azadirachta indica A. Juss) leaf extract against group B coxsackieviruses. J Commun Dis 1999;31(2):79−90.

[28] Bogdan C. Nitric oxide and the immune response. Nat Immunol 2001;2(10):907−16.

[29] DeGroote MA, Fang FC. Antimicrobial properties of nitric oxide. In: Fang FC, editor. Nitric Oxide and infection. New York: Kluwer Academic/Plenum Publishers; 1999. p. 231−61.

[30] Nathan C, Shiloh MU. Reactive oxygen and nitrogen intermediates in the relationship between mammalian hosts and microbial pathogens. Proc Natl Acad Sci USA 2000;97:8841−8.

[31] Bogdan C, Rollinghoff M, Diefenbach A. Reactive oxygen and reactive nitrogen intermediates in innate and specific immunity. Curr Opin Immunol 2000;12:64−76.

[32] Nathan C. Nitric oxide as a secretory product of mammalian cells. FASEB J 1992;6:3051−64.

[33] Bogdan C. The function of nitric oxide in the immune system. In: Mayer B, editor. Handbook of experimental pharmacology. Nitric Oxide. Heidelberg: Springer; 2000. p. 443−92.

[34] Xie K, Dong Z, Fidler IJ. Activation of nitric oxide gene for inhibition of cancer metastasis. J Leukoc Biol 1996;797:797−803.

[35] Pervin S, Singh R, Chaudhuri G. Nitric oxide−induced cytostasis and cell cycle arrest of a human breast cancer cell line (MDA-MB-231): potential role of cyclin D1. Proc Natl Acad Sci USA 2001;98:3583−8.

[36] Bauer PM, Fukuto JM, Pegg AE, Ignarro LJ. Nitric oxide inhibits ornithine decarboxylase via S-nitrosylation of cysteine 360 in the active site of the enzyme. J Biol Chem 2001;276:34458−64.

[37] Henson SE, Nichols TC, Holers VM, Karp DR. The ectoenzyme γ-glutamyl transpeptidase regulates antiproliferative effects of *S*-nitrosoglutathione on human T and B lymphocytes. J Immunol 1999;163:1845−52.

[38] Spiecker M, Darius H, Kaboth K, Hübner F, Liao JK. Differential regulation of endothelial cell adhesion molecule expression by nitric oxide donors and antioxidants. J Leukoc Biol 1998;63:732−9.

[39] Dalton DK, Haynes L, Chu CQ, Swain SL, Wittmer S. Interferon-γ eliminates responding CD4 T cells during mycobacterial infection by inducing apoptosis of activated CD4 T cells. J Exp Med 2000;192:117−22.

[40] Bobe P, Karim B, Danièle G, Paule O, Linda L, Roger H. Nitric oxide mediation of active immunosuppression associated with graft-versus-host reaction. Blood 1999;94:1028−37.

[41] Tarrant TK, Silver PB, Wahlsten JL, Rizzo LV, Chan CC, Wiggert B, et al. Interleukin-12 protects from a Th1-mediated autoimmune disease, experimental autoimmune uveitis, through a mechanism involving IFN-γ, nitric oxide and apoptosis. J Exp Med 1999;189:219−30.

[42] Shi FD, Flodström M, Kim SH, Pakala S, Cleary M. Control of the autoimmune response by type 2 nitric oxide synthase. J Immunol 2001;167:3000−6.

[43] Allione A, Bernabei P, Bosticardo M, Ariotti S, Forni G, Novelli F. Nitric oxide suppresses human T lymphocyte proliferation through IFN-gamma–dependent and IFN-gamma–independent induction of apoptosis. J Immuno 1999;163:4182–91.

[44] Angulo I, Federico G, José FG, Domingo G, Angeles MF, Fresno M. Nitric oxide producing CD11b + Ly-6G(Gr-1) + CD31(ER-MP12) + cells in the spleen of cyclophosphamide-treated mice: implications for T cell responses in immunosuppressed mice. Blood 2000;95:212–20.

[45] Kotikoski H, Alajuuma P, Moilanen E. Comparison of nitric oxide donors in lowering intra-ocular pressure in rabbits: role of cyclic GMP. J Ocul Pharmacol Ther 2002;18:11–23.

[46] Schuman JS, Erickson K, Nathanson JA. Nitrovasodilator effects on intraocular pressure and outflow facility in monkeys. Exp Eye Res 1994;58:99–105.

[47] Nathanson JA. Nitrovasodilators as a new class of ocular hypotensive agents. J Pharmacol Exp Ther 1992;260:956–65.

[48] Wizemann AJS, Wizemann V. Organic nitrate therapy in glaucoma. Am J Ophthalmol 1980;90:106–9.

CHAPTER 8

"Gleaming and Deadly White"[1]: Toxic Cosmetics in the Roman World

Susan Stewart

The range of cosmetic products available to the ancient Romans was extensive and included foundations, face powders, antiwrinkle creams, hair dyes, eye makeup, rouge, breath fresheners, deodorants, and hair removers.[2] Cosmetics were used largely, though not exclusively, by women who, in applying these products, endeavored to attain the perfection embodied in the literary descriptions and visual representations of fictional women, imagined goddesses, and often idealized members of the social elite. In accordance with contemporary standards, women strove to make their faces look pale with just a hint of pink, their eyes seem large, their hair an attractive color, their skin smooth and their bodies free from unwanted hair. In reality, some of the makeup applied to achieve this desired "look" not only had the potential to enhance, alter, conceal, or remove but could also be poisonous. The general vocabulary relating to makeup reflects this ambiguity; *medicamentum*, meaning cosmetics in Latin, refers not only to cosmetics and to medicines but also to poisons and even enchantments. Similarly, the Greek word *pharmakon* pertains to medicines or substances taken either inwardly in the form of oils or drafts or topically in the form of ointments, and also refers to a poisonous drug, charm or spell.[3]

The main toxic substances used in makeup, either as beauty products in their own right or as ingredients in beauty products, were the various minerals; in particular, lead, antimony, mercury, and arsenic. In this paper, I examine the facts and the fiction that surround the use of these minerals, concentrating on the period of the Roman Empire, when the expansion of Roman domination brought flourishing trade, even with

---

[1]See Nicander Alexipharmica 2.74 ff.

[2]There is no conclusive evidence that the Romans used lipstick.

[3]For *medicamentum* see Petr. 126, Ov. *AA.* 3.205 (cosmetic), Cic. Pis 6.13 (medicine), Suet. Calig. 50 (enchanted potion), Varr. Ap. Non. 345, 23Liv. 8.18. (poison). For *pharmakon* see Hes. *Op.* 485 Hom, *Il.* 4.191 (remedy), Hom. *Od.* 4.220 (magic potion), *Th.* 2.48 (poison), Emp. 23.3 (color, paint).

History of Toxicology and Environmental Health. DOI: http://dx.doi.org/10.1016/B978-0-12-801506-3.00008-X

countries beyond the borders of the Roman Empire, and encouraged familiarity not only with the actual ingredients or products themselves but also with the ideas and practices of other cultures in respect of cosmetics.

A good part of our scientific or quasi-scientific information relating to the Romans' use and understanding of these dangerous substances comes from the *Historia Naturalis*, the encyclopedic work of Pliny the Elder; note that, in turn, some of his knowledge was gleaned from the *Materia Medica* of the Greek physician Dioscurides. There are a number of medical texts, written not only in Greek (as much medical learning was Greek in origin and many in the profession were Greek) but also in Latin, that make reference to makeup; for example, the works of Galen, Scribonius Largus and Celsus. Other writers, from the Satirists (Juvenal, for instance) to the love poets (among them, Ovid and Propertius) and indeed the dramatists (Plautus and Terence) include references to makeup as a matter of social comment and a vehicle for humor. That is to say, nonmedical writers often included references to cosmetics in their text because this topic was a useful rhetorical tool for the purposes of defining the feminine and at the same time defaming the character of men. Moreover, to all intents and purposes, the literary evidence we have for cosmetics was penned by men, which contributed to gender bias and denied women, who used cosmetics most, a voice. In tackling the subject of ancient cosmetics, scholars must appreciate the importance of the literary rhetoric while, at same time, endeavoring to separate the fact (where that is possible) from the fiction. On the plus side, however, there is plenty of written material to work with, indicating familiarity with makeup both on the part of the writer and that of his audience.

Aside from the literary evidence, an abundance of visual images and archaeological remains survive that pertain to the matter of cosmetics. Contemporary artwork, including paintings, mosaics, sculptures and funerary reliefs, also reflect familiarity with beauty products. Note, however, that there are plenty of rhetorical messages (relating to wealth, status and gender, for example) here too. Women are depicted at their toilette with all the paraphernalia that making up entailed; servants, mirrors, boxes, bottles, palettes, mixing spoons, and the rest.[4] There is, however, virtually nothing among the surviving images that can be said categorically to show women actually wearing makeup.

[4]See for example Ref. [1] fig 30.

Furthermore, men do not appear anywhere in the visual record associated with cosmetics. Turning to the archaeological evidence, the pots (*pyxides*) and bottles (*unguentaria*) that contained beauty products in use at this time survive in abundance. Where we are lucky enough to find some residue inside these vessels, this can now be analyzed using modern noninvasive techniques including synchrotron radiation and mass spectrometry [2].

Ancient cosmetics is an area of study that, until relatively recently, merited scant attention; it was given little if any space, in scholarly books where the topic might have been relevant and somewhat more attention in books for the general reader, where inaccurate information was often reiterated again and again by different authors, thereby allowing fiction to appear as fact. However, due to the influence of feminism and an increasing interest in gender studies, some valuable work has been done on makeup in the last few decades; for example, the work of Olson, Wyke, and Richlin on gender and makeup, on the rhetoric surrounding cosmetics, and on the nature of the substances themselves.[5] Having made these points as regards research into ancient cosmetics in general, in this paper I move on to discuss toxic cosmetics specifically.

8.1 A FAIR COMPLEXION

> Psmithium, *also that is* cerussa, *or lead acetate is produced at lead works* ...*it is useful for giving women a fair complexion.*
> *(Pliny the Elder HN 34.176)*

White lead (*cerussa* in Latin, in Greek *pysmithion*) was manufactured in the classical period by steeping lead shavings in vinegar. Women applied the resultant white powder to make their faces appear pale, a matter not only of fashion, but also of status. A pale complexion could suggest to the onlooker that the individual upon whom he or she had settled his or her gaze did not spend too much time outside; that is, she was not a working-class woman but instead belonged to the upper echelons of Roman society. Equally, a pale complexion could imply that the woman sporting it was healthy, fertile, and

[5]For a general introduction to the topic of Roman cosmetics see Ref. [3]. For work on the nature of cosmetic products themselves (from a historian's point of view) see Ref. [4]. Also Ref. [5]. For gender matters and the discourse of rhetoric and reality in respect of cosmetics see Ref. [6]. Also Ref. [7].

therefore likely to make a good marriage partner. While exposure to lead has a cumulative effect corroding the surface of the skin as well as causing potential damage to the central nervous system and to the main internal organs, lead poisoning can also result in infertility; so much for the assumption that a pale complexion might indicate success in producing a healthy son and heir.

Although there were certainly safer foundations on the market, including, for example, kaolin (*creta*) and "white earths" such as *chia terra*, white lead (*cerussa*) is most popularly referred to in the written texts. However, to what extent white lead was used as makeup compared with any other substance applied for the same purpose in the Roman world remains unknown. In the archaeological record, finds of white lead are not uncommon. Lumps of white lead have been found in cosmetic boxes excavated from graves in cemeteries in Corinth that date from the Hellenistic period [8]. However, samples found at Pompeii (and therefore dating from the first century AD), as well as samples from other sites in the west dating from the Roman period, show a prevalence for more natural chalk-based alternatives [9].

Although this data is fascinating, there is little we can draw from it in terms of the scale of use at any particular time. Nor indeed can we establish any preference for applying a particular product. In short, we cannot assume, on the basis of the analysis of some samples whose survival is, after all, pure chance, that by the time of the Roman Empire white lead was being rejected in favor of other substances.

What we do know is that those in the medical profession, including Celsus and Galen, along with Pliny the Elder and others with some medical knowledge, were aware of the dangers of lead. While Celsus expounds on the healing properties of this substance, as a treatment for wounds, headaches and joint pain, for example, he includes remedies to counteract its poison too.[6] Pliny also acknowledges that while *cerussa* "is useful for giving women a fair complexion it is a deadly poison" (Plin. *HN* 34.176). Vitruvius, writing about the use of lead in a wider context, that is, as a building material, also notes that "cerussite in particular is said to be injurious to the human system" (Vit. *De Arch.* 8.6.10–11).

---

[6]2.42.166 (wounds); 1.272, 1.458 (headache and joint pain) and requiring an antidote 2.122.

Although awareness of these hazards is clearly expressed in some of the written texts, we cannot be sure how far the general public understood the dangers of lead. Poets and playwrights, Martial and Plautus, for example, concentrate on putting across the rhetorical message that wearing makeup reflects the immorality of the wearer and his or her lack of status, rather than referring to the dangerous nature of particular cosmetics. In love poetry, drama, and satirical verse, it is often old women who are noted as wearing white lead to conceal their wrinkles, the telltale signs of aging; this was part of the rhetoric portraying women as devious characters while also stressing the unattractiveness of old age. It is interesting to speculate that, in the case of some women at least, the appearance of age might have been as much the result of the toxic effects of wearing lead makeup as it was a true reflection of advancing years, though this is impossible to verify.

Early in the twentieth century, scholars argued that lead poisoning was a significant factor in the collapse of the Roman Empire. This theory was based on the belief that exposure to lead resulted in infertility and a falling birth rate among the Roman aristocracy. The argument in favor of this theory reemerged in 1983, expounded by geochemist Jerome Nriagu [10]. It is certainly true that the people of the Roman world, in particular those living in the cities across the Empire, would have been exposed to lead in many areas of their lives. Not only did they apply lead as a cosmetic, but also their water supply flowed through lead pipes. They cooked in lead vessels, applied plasters containing lead for medical purposes, and even ingested lead in their wine, where it was used as a preservative. However, with the exception of one possible rather earlier account of lead poisoning noted by the Greek poet Nicander, writing in the second century BC, together with evidence of relatively high lead levels found in exhumed bones from the Roman period, we have no definite record of lead poisoning until the seventh century AD.[7] The theory that lead poisoning contributed significantly to the collapse of the Roman Empire is largely discredited by scholars today, and the scale of the health impact from the use of lead argued for in earlier research is believed to have been overestimated. Indeed, when Nriagu raised these theories in the 1980s they were quickly refuted by Scarborough, an eminent classicist and pharmacologist [11]. In dismissing this argument here, I point out that

[7]Nicander *Alexipharmica* 1.600. Paulus of Aegina 3.64.

exposure to lead through cosmetics was but a small part of the ancients' contact with this potentially dangerous substance.

8.2 ROUGE

She's blushing!—Yes, modesty suits a pale skin but it is better put on. The real thing can be a nuisance.

(Ov. Am. 3.7.7)

Not only white but also red pigments, such as red lead or lead tetroxide (*minium*), were used as makeup. These were applied as rouge. Cinnabar (*cinnibaris*) from red mercuric sulfide, another brilliant red, was also used to heighten the color of the cheeks and create a complexion that could be compared to the subtle colors of nature. The poet Ovid describes the ideal female complexion as follows: "In her face the lily and the rose are glowing still—snow white, pale red" (Ov. *Am* 3.35–6).

Both red lead and cinnabar were known poisons at this time. Indeed, inhaling the dust or powder from these beauty products may have been a potential health hazard not only for the women wearing these cosmetics but also for the maidservants tasked with applying them. Cheaper and safer alternatives did exist; for example, the dregs of red wine *(faex)*, the red dye extracted from the roots of alkanet (*anchusa*), a type of borage, and the juice of the mulberry (*morum*). According to Ovid, one woman even rubbed her cheeks with poppies steeped in cold water.[8]

What, then, was the appeal of known dangerous substances such as red lead and cinnabar? As with white lead, we do not know how far the general populace were aware of the dangers of these substances; some may have used them unaware of the health hazards. However, I offer an alternative explanation. Red lead was imported (largely from Spain) and cinnabar brought to the cities of the Mediterranean from Spain and India. Red pigments such as these, sometimes coming from beyond the boundaries of the known world in antiquity, were commonly believed to be the congealed blood of dragons. The far-flung origins of these rouges and the stories that built up around them gave these products considerable exotic appeal. Their exclusivity, even scarcity when compared with the rather more readily available supply

[8]Ov. *De Med. Fac.* 100.

of leftover wine or mulberries, bestowed on the owner and user both glamour and status. The pursuit of this illusion of grandeur, if you like, imparted by the enthusiastic use of such mysterious products as red lead and cinnabar might have encouraged the use of these substances, overriding any consideration of their dangers.

8.3 EYE MAKEUP

In the same mines as silver there is found what is properly to be described as a stone, made of white and shiny but not transparent froth; several names are used for it, stimi, stibi, alabastrum *and sometimes* larbasis

(Plin. HN 33.101).

Powdered antimony sulfide, another toxic substance, which not only was toxic when ingested but also dangerous when absorbed through the skin, had been a popular black eye makeup used for brows and lashes and to define eyes since ancient Egyptian times; the Egyptians called this *mesdemet*. Both Dioscorides and Pliny the Elder describe antimony (*stimmi* or *stibium*) as an eye cosmetic. According to the former, "*stimmi* was 'a good paste of stibnite is a cosmetic'... enlarger of the eyes" (Dios. 1. 555). Pliny the Elder noted that "Antimony has astringent and cooling properties but is chiefly used for the eyes ... in beauty washes for women's eyebrows it has the property of magnifying the eyes" (Plin. *HN* 33.102). An eye makeup known as *fuligo*, consisting, in safe form, of either of soot or lampblack, could also be manufactured in a potentially harmful variety from powdered antimony. *Galena*, another eye makeup used from ancient Egyptian times, was poisonous even to the touch. Made from malachite, a lead ore, mixed with silver, galena was also applied in powdered form. Soot (*favilla*), no doubt a cheaper and much less prestigious option in terms of eye makeup, was easily obtainable from the spitting oil lamps common to the city's brothels and, by implication and on account of its ready availability, probably used by lower-class women.

Eye makeup, whether powdered antimony, soot, or *galena*, was applied much like modern-day eyeliner and mascara and, for ease of application, could be mixed with water or perhaps scented oil such as oil of roses. In the archaeological record, eye makeup containers often consist of two tubes joined together. One would have held the powdered antimony or lampblack and the other the liquid, either water or oil, for mixing. The addition of scented oil might have added to the attractiveness of eye makeup (in terms of smell), though of course if it were based on antimony, such a mixture would be no less toxic.[9]

The frequency with which archaeologists come across oculists' stamps attests to the proliferation of eye diseases at this time. Eye infections were caused by a number of factors including heat and dust as well as by a lack of understanding as to how bacteria spread. Some of the treatments prescribed for eye complaints contained some of the same toxic ingredients as (or were the same as) toxic products that were applied as makeup. A lead sulfide mixture known as *collyrium* was recognized as an eye salve with healing properties; the term *collyrium* also was used as a general term for eyeliner. Recent research has established that in fact eye makeup containing lead, mercury, or lead compounds was not all bad news.[10] Indeed, these products may have had an antibacterial effect, and basing our evidence on the use of these substances, it would appear the ancients understood these benefits.

8.4 HAIR REMOVERS

How nearly was I recommending to you that there should be no shocking goat in the armpits and that your legs should not be rough with harsh hair.
(Ov. Ars. Am. 3.194)

In classical antiquity, underarm hair was taboo for both sexes, being associated with bad odor and poor hygiene. Pumice stone was used for removing unwanted hair. Tweezers too served this purpose and are common site finds from this period. As an abundance of these tools have been excavated at army camps where the community would have been predominantly male, we can safely conclude, especially given the accepted code regarding body hair at this time, that men did indeed use these toilet instruments to remove hair. According to Seneca, hair plucking was a service available to men when they visited the public baths.[11] At that time, the ideal was that the entire surface of women's bodies should be hairless. The use of depilatory creams and pastes was associated predominantly with the removal of hair from the

---

[9]Juv. 2.93. Juvenal gives us an acutely observed description of a transvestite applying soot with a damp pin.
[10]Cf. [12]. See also Ref. [13].
[11]Sen. Ep. 56.2.

female body. However, Pliny the Elder does claim to be "ashamed to confess that the chief value now set on resin is for a depilatory for men" (Plin. *HN* 24. 124).[12]

While using a pumice stone or pulling one's hair out with a set of tweezers was essentially safe and effective even if it might have irritated the surface of the skin, depilatory pastes included some toxic concoctions, in particular arsenic (*arsenicum*). There was also the option of orpiment (*auripigmentum*)—yellow arsenic—the stuff, when it came to murder by poisoning, of the modern detective novel. Furthermore, one might apply *psilothrum*, a toxic mixture of arsenic and quicklime that was green in color.[13] Antimony was also an ingredient in hair removers. Some, like orpiment, were believed to have a cleansing effect.[14] Pliny confuses us when it comes to how some of these substances might have worked, stating that "before using any depilatory the hairs must first be pulled out" (Plin. *HN* 32.137). It is possible that these concoctions were intended to stop the hair growing in again rather than to remove the surface hair there already. Certainly, most of these products were not only toxic but also caustic; the astringent qualities of such products would have stripped off skin as well as hair if left on for any length of time.

To conclude, some ancient cosmetics were indeed potentially dangerous, especially if used regularly over a prolonged length of time. In practical terms, without any contemporary record of extensive poisoning as a result of using these products, we cannot draw any real conclusions as to the how these risks materialized. We do know that the ancients continued to use such products despite at least some knowledge of the dangers. Perhaps we can liken this usage to our own predisposition to smoke despite being aware of the damage this can cause to our health. So, where the dangers were understood, the ideological message, that is, the exclusive status bestowed on the individual female through the use and ownership of specific beauty products, may have been encouragement enough to take the risk. The flip side of this argument might be that, rhetorically speaking, these substances could be seen to poison woman as a gender, corrupting her physical

---

[12]Note also his remark that "Depilatories I myself indeed regard them as a woman's cosmetic, but now today men also use them" (Plin. *HN* 26.164).

[13]Mart. 6.93.

[14]Celsus 5.5.

morality in their application and mirroring her innermost flaws. However, those who condemned cosmetics outright (satirists and some poets and playwrights) do not dwell on the reality of the poisonous nature of these substances. Certainly, in order to gain any sense of reality *vis-à-vis* the use of harmful beauty products by the Romans we need to treat the evidence very carefully, teasing any suggestion of real life from the rhetorical message to which this subject matter is so firmly attached. However, it is the rhetoric that in a sense is a clue to the reality surrounding the use of toxic makeup at this time. That is to say, the scholar must understand that the rhetoric surrounding cosmetics was also among the reasons for their use.

REFERENCES

[1] Allason-Jones L. Women in Roman Britain. London: British Museum Press; 1989. p. 92 fig. 30.

[2] Ribechini E, Modugno F, Perez-Arantegui J, Columbini MP. Discovering the composition of ancient cosmetics and remedies: analytical techniques and materials. Anal Bioanal Chem 2011;401(6):1727−38.

[3] Stewart S. Cosmetics and perfumes in the Roman world. Stroud: Tempus; 2007.

[4] Olson K. Cosmetics in Roman antiquity: substance, remedy, poison. Class World 2009;102 (3):291−310.

[5] Stewart S. Cosmetics and perfumes in the Roman world: a glossary. In: Harlow M, editor. Dress and identity. Oxford: British Archaeological Reports; 2012.

[6] Wyke M. Woman in a mirror: the rhetoric of adornment in the Roman world. In: Archer L, Fichler S, Wyke M, editors. Women in ancient societies: an illusion of the night. London/ New York: Macmillan; 1994. p. 134−51.

[7] Richlin A. Making up a woman: the face of Roman gender. In: Eilberg Schwartz H, Doniger W, editors. Off with her head: the denial of women's identity in myth religion and culture. California/Berkeley: University of California Press; 1995.

[8] Shear TL. Psmythion. In: Shear TL, editor. Classical studies presented to Edward Capps. Princeton, NJ: Princeton University Press; 1936. p. 314−7.

[9] Welcomme E, Walter P, Van Elslande E, Tsoucaris G. Investigation of white pigments used as make-up during the Greco-Roman period. Appl Phys A 2006;83(4):551−6.

[10] Nriagu J. Lead and lead poisoning in antiquity. N Engl J Med 1983;308:660−3.

[11] Scarborough J. The myth of lead poisoning among the Romans: an essay review. J Hist Med 1984;39:469−75.

[12] Murube J. Ocular cosmetics in ancient times. Ocul Surf 2013;11(1):2−7.

[13] Tapsoba I, Arbault S, Walter P, Amatore C. Finding out Egyptian Gods' secret using analytical chemistry biomedical properties of Egyptian black makeup revealed by amperometry at single cells. J Anal Chem 2010;82(2):457−60.

CHAPTER 9

Poisonous Medicine in Ancient China

Yan Liu

> *For all things under the heaven, nothing is more vicious than the poison of aconite. Yet a good doctor packs and stores it, because it is useful.*
>
> **Masters of Huainan (second century BCE)**

The standard Chinese word for poison is *du* 毒. Modern readers often frown upon the word, because it invites associations with danger, harm, and intrigue. But this translation is misleading, as *du* in the past had diverse, even opposite meanings. At the core of them lay the notion of potency, the ability not just to harm as a poison but also to cure as a medicine. Accordingly, instead of avoiding poisons entirely, classical Chinese medicine strategically utilized them for therapy. This article will probe the roots of this important pharmacological tradition in ancient China. The history of Chinese medicine cannot ignore the history of poison.

9.1 ETYMOLOGY OF *DU*

Let us start with the first dictionary of Chinese history, *Explaining and Analyzing Characters* (*Shuowen jiezi*), compiled in 100 CE. The dictionary explains the basic meaning of *du* as thickness, which refers to the physical shape of mountains. Thickness implies heaviness, abundance, and potency; the word does not carry a negative sense.

Further study of the scripts of *du* reveals conflicting implications. Two Han dynasty (206 BCE—220 CE) variants of *du* are shown in Figure 9.1 [1]. The two scripts share the upper part of the character *tu* 土, which means soil, and relatedly, growth. The lower parts of the two differ. In the first variant, it is written as *wu* 毋, which means stop. In the second, we see a different character, *mu* 母, which means mother, and implicitly, nurture. Therefore, depending on how the lower part is written, *du* signifies either prohibiting or promoting growth. Thickness could elicit opposite outcomes.

History of Toxicology and Environmental Health. DOI: http://dx.doi.org/10.1016/B978-0-12-801506-3.00009-1

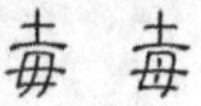

Figure 9.1 Two variants of du in the Han.

9.2 *DU* IN CHINESE PHARMACOLOGY

How do these two meanings manifest themselves in ancient Chinese pharmacology? Let us examine the first drug treatise in China, *Divine Farmer's Classic of Materia Medica* (*Shennong bencao jing*), compiled during the first century CE by the Han officials who specialized in drugs. It names 365 drugs, and parses them into three groups. Drugs in the top tier are considered nontoxic (*wudu*), and are supposed to lighten the body, supplement *qi*, avert aging, and prolong life; drugs in the middle tier, defined as either nontoxic or toxic (*youdu*), can prevent maladies and replenish depletions; drugs in the bottom tier, most of which are toxic, effectively cure illnesses [2, pp. 23–25].

Here we see two key features of Chinese pharmacology. First, drugs are categorized and defined by their toxicity or *du*. This *du*-centered grouping of drugs would remain fundamental to Chinese medicine throughout the premodern period. Second, toxicity figures not as something to be avoided at all costs, but as potency valuable in the cure of illnesses. At the same time, the text also notes the danger of toxic drugs, warning that one should only use them temporarily and cautiously. A toxic substance is a double-edged sword; it cures if handled properly, and harms if it is not.

What, then, is the proper use of a toxic drug? The *Divine Farmer's Classic* specifies two keys.

First is dosage control. The text declares that when ingesting a toxic drug, one should start with a dose as small as a millet seed. If this proves insufficient, one should increase the dosage gradually until the patient is cured. The amount of the drug, in short, has to be carefully calibrated to the patient's state of recovery.

Second is drug combination. Chinese pharmacy frequently combines drugs to maximize their remedial power. The *Divine Farmer's Classic* defines six ways of combination, ranging from mutual facilitation to mutual annihilation. Relevant to the use of toxic materials is the strategy of "mutual inhibition" (*xiangwei*), which adds a nontoxic drug to a toxic one to curb its potency, yet preserve its therapeutic efficacy.

Although toxic substances are powerful medicines, the *Divine Farmer's Classic* places most of them in the bottom tier, regarding them as inferior to nontoxic ones in the middle and top tiers. Rather than treating illnesses, drugs in the middle tier aim to strengthen the body to keep one healthy. This fits well with a medical philosophy prominent at the time, manifested by the Han dynasty medical classic, *Yellow Emperor's Inner Classic* (*Huangdi neijing*): It is better to prevent illnesses from occurring than to cure them after they arise [3, p. 57].

Furthermore, drugs in the top tier, all nontoxic, target a higher goal of longevity, which resonates with the Chinese ideal of "nourishing life" (*yangsheng*). This ancient tradition proposed regular ingestion of tonic substances (mushrooms, resin, mica, etc.) combined with gymnastics, breathing, and meditation techniques to enhance life [4]. All these methods aimed to purify the body and eliminate toxic substances that triggered its decay. Nontoxic drugs for "nourishing life," therefore, induce an opposite bodily effect to that of toxic ones: The former promote purification to "lighten the body" by releasing its toxic burden, whereas the latter, with their characteristic "thickness," invigorate the body to combat maladies. Understanding *du* in this context allows us to appreciate its paradoxical meaning in Chinese medicine: A toxic drug effectively cures illnesses, but impedes one from achieving a higher goal—the cultivation of the body to attain a healthy, long life.

9.3 ACONITE, THE POWER TO CURE

We have explored thus far the principle underlying the use of toxic drugs in ancient China. Let us now consider a specific example, aconite, one of the most commonly used drugs in Chinese medicine. Aconite encompasses a group of herbs of the *Aconitum* species that Chinese sources refer to by a variety of names (*fuzi, wutou, tianxiong, wuhui, jin*, etc.). In general, these names correspond to different parts of the herb, or parts collected in different seasons. For example, *wutou* refers to the parental tuber of the herb harvested in the spring, whereas *fuzi*, which literally means "attached offspring," depicts the daughter tuber that grows in the summer. Chinese pharmacology attributes distinct medicinal functions to each of these varieties of aconite [5, pp. 91–143].

More than 50 species of aconite are utilized in Chinese medicine today, with *Aconitum carmichaeli* from northern Sichuan (southwest China) as the major production. According to modern pharmacology, the main toxic component in aconite is aconitine-type alkaloid: 0.2 mg of it, taken orally, suffices to poison a person, while 3−5 mg may cause death by cardiovascular and neurological failure. When administered in smaller doses, however, aconitine and other alkaloids in the herb can relieve pain, reduce inflammation, and strengthen the heart [6]. The use of aconite, therefore, becomes the art of moderating the herb's toxicity while preserving its therapeutic power.

Early evidence for the medicinal use of aconite in China comes from a collection of medical recipes excavated from Mawangdui in modern Hunan (southern China), which date from the second century BCE in the early years of the Western Han dynasty (206 BCE−9 CE). Among the over 400 substances in these recipes, aconite was the second most-used drug (21 times), only surpassed by cinnamon. In most cases, aconite was applied externally, often mixed with other drugs, to treat wounds, abscess, scabies, and itch. When taken internally, it acted as a tonic to replenish *qi*, boost sexual energy, and prolong life. In addition, several recipes also employed aconite to achieve speed of travel, evincing its magical power [7].

Aconite remained popular in the following centuries, but its functions altered. During the Eastern Han dynasty (25−220 CE), the herb was harnessed mainly as an internal medicine to treat cold illnesses, whereas its tonic and magical activities receded. The influential medical work *Treatise on Cold Damage Disorders* (*Shanghan lun*), compiled by Zhang Zhongjing in the early third century, used aconite frequently; we find the drug in 20% of all recipes (23 in number) [8]. Conspicuously, these recipes always mixed aconite with other herbs, most often licorice and ginger, which echoes the strategy of drug combination to mitigate toxicity mentioned earlier. Moreover, most recipes employed processed aconite, the product of roasting the herb or soaking it in water. These methods effectively reduce toxicity, as modern tests show that they trigger the physical loss and hydrolysis of alkaloids in the herb. Crude aconite was still used in some recipes but mainly for medical emergencies.

What is the therapeutic rationale of using this toxic drug in Chinese medicine? The *Divine Farmer's Classic* defines aconite as a warming drug, which, according to the principle of opposites, treats cold ailments.

The symptoms include wind-induced coldness, coughing, pain in the joints, and blood clotting. Aconite, with its heating power, can dissipate cold and break up stagnation in the body. This process often generates strong, if not traumatic, bodily sensations. Zhang Zhongjing, for instance, noted that after patients took one dose of an aconite decoction, their body had a condition of impediment; after three doses, they became dizzy. Zhang, however, did not treat these reactions as pathologies, but rather as positive signs of the drug's efficacy. This interpretation expresses the core philosophy of deploying toxic drugs in ancient China, aptly summarized by an aphorism—If a drug does not deliver a spell of dizziness, it cannot cure severe illnesses.

9.4 ACONITE, THE POWER TO KILL

Now that we have reviewed the medicinal use of aconite, we will turn to its sinister functions. In fact, before becoming a medicine, aconite had long been used to kill. The earliest evidence comes from a fourth-century BCE text, *Discourses of the States* (*Guoyu*), where the herb appeared in a court murder. In 656 BCE, Li Ji, a concubine of Duke Xian of the Jin state, planned a conspiracy to remove the heir apparent, Shen Sheng, so her own son could succeed to the throne. She asked Shen Sheng to offer food to his father, but beforehand secretly added aconite (*jin*) into the meat. When the Duke was about to eat the food, Li Ji asked him to first test it on a dog, which died instantly. Seeing himself in trouble, Shen Sheng fled away, and later committed suicide.

Six centuries later, during the Han dynasty, aconite figured in another court murder. According to a second-century CE source, *History of the Western Han* (*Hanshu*), in 71 BCE Huo Xian, the wife of a powerful general, planned to murder the Empress Xu to seize the position for her daughter. She hired a court physician named Chunyu Yan to present medicine to the empress, who had just given birth to a child. Chunyu Yan mixed aconite (*fuzi*) in the medicine, and persuaded the empress to take it for recovering from childbirth. The empress died soon after. The murder was ingenious, covered by the reality that women often died after delivery at the time. Intriguingly, after the empress ingested some of the "medicine," she complained that her head felt dizzy, wondering whether she was poisoned. Chunyu Yan claimed that the effect was normal for healing, and convinced her to take more, leading to her death. The line between medicine and poison is thin; so is that between life and death [9].

In addition to being favored for murder, aconite was also employed in hunting and warfare, mainly as an arrow poison. The dictionary *Explaining and Analyzing Characters* includes a pre-Han script of *du* with a radical that signifies knife. This ancient form of *du* implies its association with weapons, possibly coated with poison for hunting or military purposes. This may be the original function of poison in China. Aconite as arrow poison is suggested by one of its many names—*shewang*, which means "shoot and ensnare." We find evidence for this function in a medical manuscript from Mawangdui (second century BCE), which includes seven recipes to treat aconite (*wuhui*) poisoning. One of them prescribed applying a few herbs onto the wound, which was likely caused by arrow poison [7, p. 238]. The example indicates that by the second century BCE, the use of aconite-coated arrows was so prevalent that an antidote had been developed.

Finding antidotes went hand in hand with making poisons. Among its six drug combinations, the *Divine Farmer's Classic* specifies one as "mutual annihilation" (*xiangsha*), in which one drug is harnessed as antidote to counter the other as poison. Some oft-used antidotes in Chinese medicine were licorice, ginseng, ginger, honey, and salt. To counteract aconite poisoning, soybean soup was the primary choice in antiquity. Modern studies indicate that the rich proteins in soybean can coat and precipitate toxic materials in the body, explaining its antidotal efficacy. Not surprisingly, many of these antidotes, such as licorice and ginger, overlap with those that mitigate toxic drugs by "mutual inhibition," discussed earlier. Dosage is probably the determining factor that allows the same substance to act in these two distinct manners.

9.5 FROM *DU* TO *PHARMAKON*

Thus far we have examined how *du* in Chinese pharmacology ambiguously straddled medicine and poison. This duality, of course, was not unique to China. The English word pharmacy, derives from the Greek word *pharmakon*, which means both remedy and poison. The use of toxic materials in Greek medicine had already appeared in the Hippocratic Corpus (fifth or fourth century BCE), which frequently prescribed a herb called hellebore. The herb served as a strong purgative to treat humoral imbalance, gynecological disorders, and pulmonary illnesses, almost reaching the status of a panacea. On the other hand, the Hippocratic writers observed the harmful, even lethal effects of hellebore when administered carelessly [10].

We encounter more toxic drugs in Dioscorides' *De materia medica*, a monumental work in Western pharmacology compiled in the first century CE [11]. Dioscorides discussed many toxic substances in his treatise, which can be divided into two groups. The first group contained about 50 drugs that produced unpleasant but mild side effects such as headache, dim-sightedness, and stomach discomfort. In the second group, we find a dozen drugs with stronger toxicity, including opium poppy, henbane, thorn apple, mandrake, and hemlock, the last of which was presumably the deadly poison that Socrates drank. Dosage was the key to administering these drugs; Dioscorides repeatedly warned that consuming them in excess could harm and even kill. Evidently, the therapeutic use of toxic materials is prominent in ancient Greek pharmacology.

This continuity between medicine and poison, evinced by *pharmakon*, parallels the Chinese concept of *du*. If we look further, however, we detect a subtle yet visible change in Greek pharmacology that began to distinguish poison from medicine. As early as the third century BCE, Apollodorus wrote a treatise on poison, which has been lost. Some of his toxicological knowledge was preserved a century later in Nicander's two poems, *Theriaca* and *Alexipharmaca*. The poems, arguably the earliest toxicological writing in Greek antiquity, offered detailed accounts of poisonous animals and plants as well as poison-induced symptoms [12]. Nicander's poems were highly influential because later authors, including the famous Roman physician Galen, extensively cited him as a source on toxicology.

The separation of poison from medicine became more patent in *De materia medica*. Although Dioscorides utilized many toxic materials for therapy, he also identified some poisons in which he discerned no medicinal value, such as wolfsbane, yew, and meadow saffron. He listed these poisons simply to warn against them. Despite the blurred boundary between medicine and poison in Greek antiquity, then, a group of toxic substances began to gradually move out of the *pharmakon* continuum. This separation became more pronounced in medieval Europe. In China, however, we do not see a similar phenomenon. All drugs in Chinese pharmacy, including highly toxic ones, were perceived to have medicinal value; no absolute poisons existed. This does not mean that toxicological knowledge was absent in ancient China. Quite the contrary, we find abundant discussions about poisons, poisoning, and antidotes, as shown above. Yet in classical Chinese medicine, toxicology was always part of pharmacology.

No example better illustrates this divergence than the distinct fates of aconite in Greek and Chinese medicine. In *De materia medica* the herb, there called wolfsbane, was only used as a poison to kill wolves, without any perceived curative functions. Correspondingly, the first-century CE Roman naturalist Pliny the Elder called the herb "plant arsenic," evoking its harmful nature. But in China, as we have seen, aconite was highly valued for its therapeutic power, hailed as the "chief of hundreds of drugs." This marked difference points to diverging philosophies of utilizing toxic substances between Greek and Chinese pharmacology. If we compare Dioscorides' comments on the side effects of toxic drugs to the aforementioned Chinese aphorism that if a drug does not cause dizziness, it cannot cure severe illnesses, this much seems clear: Greek medicine prescribed drugs in spite of their toxicity; Chinese medicine, because of it.

The prominent use of poisons as curative agents in Chinese history urges us to rethink the principles and practices of Chinese medicine today. Contemporary views of classical Chinese medicine often contrast the benign naturalness of Chinese herbal remedies with the dangerous side effects of Western synthetic drugs. This dichotomy is misconceived. It not only overlooks the abundant poisons in Chinese pharmacy but also, at a fundamental level, fails to understand the paradoxical nature of drug therapy. We take drugs to cure disease or remain healthy, yet for any drug we consume, be it aconite or aspirin, ginseng or vitamin, we introduce a foreign agent—hence, in a broad sense, poison—to our body. A drug's potentials for curing and harming are always intertwined. It is ultimately not the substance itself, but *how* we use it that matters. We cannot avoid poisons, for the art of medicine is the art of poison.

REFERENCES

[1] Shi ZC. Zhongguo gudai duzi jiqi xiangguan cihui kao [A study of the character *du* and related words in ancient China]. Dulixue shi yanjiu wenji [Research papers on the history of toxicology] 2004;3:1−9, [in Chinese].

[2] Unschuld PU. Medicine in China: a history of pharmaceutics. Berkeley, CA: University of California Press; 1986.

[3] Huang Di nei jing su wen: an annotated translation of Huang Di's inner classic—basic questions. [Unschuld PU and Tessenow H in collaboration with Zheng JS, Trans.]. Berkeley, CA: University of California Press; 2011.

[4] Sakade Y. Chūgoku shisō kenkyū: Iyaku yōsei, kagaku shisō hen [Studies on Chinese thought: Medicine, nourishing life, and scientific thought]. Osaka: Kansai daigaku shuppanbu; 1999, [in Japanese].

[5] Obringer F. L'aconit et l'orpiment: drogues et poisons en Chine ancienne et médiévale [Aconite and orpiment: drugs and poisons in ancient and medieval China]. Paris: Fayard; 1997, [in French].

[6] Bisset NG. Arrow poisons in China. Part II. Aconitum—botany, chemistry, and pharmacology. J Ethnopharmacol 1981;4:247–336.

[7] Harper DJ. Early Chinese medical literature: the Mawangdui medical manuscripts. London/New York: Kegan Paul International Press; 1998.

[8] Zhang ZJ. Shang Han Lun: on cold damage [Mitchell C, Feng Y, Wiseman N, Trans.]. Brookline, MA: Paradigm Publications; 1999.

[9] Li JM. Nüyi sha'ren: Xihan xupingjun huanghou mousha'an xinkao [Killing by a female physician: a new study on the murder of the Empress Xu in the Western Han]. In: Li JM, editor. Lüxingzhe de shixue [Out of place: travels throughout Chinese medical history]. Taipei: Yunchen wenhua shiye gufen youxian gongsi; 2011. p. 285–324, [in Chinese].

[10] Girard MC. L'hellébore: panacée ou placébo? [Hellebore: Panacea or placebo?]. In: Potter P, Maloney G, Désautels J, editors. La malade et les maladies dans la Collection hippocratique [The patient and the illnesses in the Hippocratic collection]. Québec: Editions du Sphinx; 1990. p. 393–405, [in French].

[11] Dioscorides P. De materia medica [Beck LY, Trans.]. Hildesheim/New York: Olms-Weidmann; 2011.

[12] Scarborough J. Nicander's toxicology I: snakes. Pharm Hist 1977;19:3–23, [Nicander's toxicology II: spiders, scorpions, insects, and myriapods. Pharm Hist 1979;21:3–34].

CHAPTER 10

The Venomous Virgin: Fact or Fantasy?

Michael Slouber

The motif of the venomous virgin, the poison damsel, or the maiden assassin who kills with her poisonous kiss became wildly popular in Europe starting around the twelfth century, and its origin can ultimately be traced back to India over 2,000 years ago. The idea is that a certain unscrupulous king might feed a young girl tolerably minute, but gradually increasing, amounts of poison or snake venom, and that by the time she was an attractive young woman, the level of toxin in her body would be so high that she could be sent to an enemy king as a gift. Upon kissing her, making love to her, or even just sharing a glass of wine with her, he would instantly fall dead.

The earliest reference to this motif is in an ancient compendium on the Indian system of medicine called Ayurveda, literally "The Science of Long-life." Written in Sanskrit in the early centuries BC, the *Suśrutasaṃhitā* is a text that focuses on surgery, but also includes a substantial book on toxicology dealing with everything from plant poisons and snakebite medicine to rabies, scorpion sting, and venomous spider bites [1]. The venomous virgin (*viṣakanyā*) is referred to in a passage on protecting a king from assassination attempts. I translate:

> *Devious enemies may attempt to kill the king with poisons. Or, women sometimes try to seduce him with various poisonous love philters, playing on his desire for beautiful women. Or, occasionally, use of a poison maiden might cause the king to give up his vital breaths. Therefore, a doctor must constantly protect the Lord of Men from poison.*
>
> Suśrutasaṃhitā 5.1.6–7

Several hundred years later, the first literary reference to the venomous virgin is in a political drama, also written in Sanskrit, by the playwright Viśākhadatta [2]. The author served the famous emperor Chandragupta II, whose name harkens back to India's first great emperor, Chandragupta Maurya. The play takes the life of the old Chandragupta as its subject, and has his wily political advisor, the

History of Toxicology and Environmental Health. DOI: http://dx.doi.org/10.1016/B978-0-12-801506-3.00010-8

famous Kautilya of Indian statecraft, manipulate his enemies to consolidate state power. According to the play, the advisor to an enemy king dispatched a poison maiden to kill the young Chandragupta, but his clever advisor Kautilya detected the plot and sent her on, untouched, as a "gift" for a third king. Incidentally, the German word for poison is *gift*, so she is a gift in both senses.

Starting sometime around the eighth or ninth century, Indian astrology gave the same name (venomous virgin, *viṣakanyā*) to an astrological condition some women were thought to have that would cause bad luck and stillborn children. This condition is still cited in Indian astrology, which remains popular even in the midst of modern technology and globalization. Such a diagnosis would spell disaster in a prospective bride's marriage arrangements, which always involves checking for astrological compatibility.

Over the centuries, the poison maiden motif must have grown in popularity in Indian story literature. Much of this early literature is lost, but vast collections of Sanskrit stories survive from as early as the twelfth century AD and attest to the motif in numerous cases. N.M. Penzer studied the story literature on poison damsels in Indian and European sources, and I will summarize his findings based on the 1952 version of his article "Poison Damsels," which was originally published in 1925 [3]. According to Penzer, one story, which recounts the same episode as the play mentioned above, has the final king killed merely by the perspiration of her hand as they walked, holding hands, around the Indian wedding fire (16). Another story uses the word "poison damsel" to refer to a cursed jewel box that causes bad luck to whomever touches it.

10.1 SECRETUM SECRETORUM

The emperor Chandragupta Maurya mentioned above, whose wise minister Kautilya supposedly saved him from a venomous virgin sent by his enemy, lived around the time Alexander the Great reached India. Although Alexander believed that he was near the end of the earth, he was forced to turn back when his troops heard about the massive armies of war elephants held by the king of India and mutinied. Legend has it that Chandragupta was a youth while Alexander was in northwestern India, that they met, and that Chandragupta learned methods of warfare from Alexander (Penzer 14).

The legend is notable because, as in the Sanskrit play about Kautilya saving Chandragupta from a venomous virgin, by the twelfth century, a similar narrative appeared for Alexander. The text was called *Secretum Secretorum* (Secret of Secrets), and while it appeared in Latin, it purported to be a translation from Arabic, itself based on a Greek original, of secret communications between Aristotle and Alexander that had been lost in antiquity. By this time, Alexander had grown incredibly popular in Europe, so the work was a sensation. It was widely accepted as authentic, was widely read, and was translated into nearly every European language. It even came to have more influence than authenticated writings about Alexander (ibid., 18). Every library in Europe has a manuscript of the *Secretum Secretorum*, and various editions and recensions developed and expanded. Some chapters even circulated as independent texts. Scholars today agree that there is no Greek original, and no proof that one ever existed (ibid., 21).

Among other fascinating stories, the work records a supposed dialogue wherein Aristotle gives advice to Alexander on how to avoid poisons. He warns him not to trust women to care for his body, and not to take medicine from a single doctor, but rather to go with the unanimous advice of several doctors. Then Aristotle reminds Alexander about the time an Indian king had dispatched a venomous virgin against him. He describes how she was fed on poison until she was like a snake, and could kill by embrace or by mere perspiration. In one Hebrew version likely to be earlier than most, Aristotle says that he fears the clever political strategists of India (ibid., 22). Like Kautilya in Chandragupta's case, Aristotle detected this threat before his protégé could fall for her. In one French version of the story, Socrates and Aristotle told two slaves to kiss the girl and they both fell down dead instantly (ibid., 25). Other versions have her kill by bite, sexual intercourse, or even just an icy glare.

Penzer notes that the Spanish author Guillem de Cervera, writing in the thirteenth century, declared that Alexander would have died if not for Aristotle's astronomical knowledge (23), and apparently Penzer has overlooked the significance of this statement. He makes passing reference to being aware of Sanskrit astrological works on this topic but dismisses them as unimportant. In fact, it seems that Guillem de Cervera had read a version of the story wherein Aristotle uses the same astrological techniques of determining a poison maiden by her horoscope to avert the attack.

Penzer describes a more elaborate fourteenth-century French rendering in which the poison girl can kill many times—a point notable to Penzer because it was emphasized in the Sanskrit play that she was a "one-time-use" weapon. Here again, I think Penzer misses the point. He seems to believe her supply of venom would be exhausted after one encounter. I believe, however, that the poison maiden was called a "one-time-use" weapon because she would be arrested and executed after the king died in her embrace.

A sixteenth-century Italian rendering that Penzer describes is even more elaborate. It has the queen of India insert a baby girl into the egg of a giant stag-eating snake, which the mother snake feeds and raises. I would interject that the Indian Rock Python does grow to 25 feet and is called *ajaga* in Sanskrit for its habit of swallowing whole goats and deer. Mother pythons do, in fact, incubate their eggs and care for their young, unlike many other Indian snakes, so the story is not so far fetched, excepting the supposed size of the egg, which is out of the question. Anyhow, in the story, the queen slowly domesticates the snake girl, who is very beautiful, and dispatches her to kill Alexander.

10.2 OTHER VERSIONS

Penzer suggests that the dispersal of the poison damsel motif was greatly enhanced by its inclusion in the *Gesta Romanorum*, a collection of stories popular among monks and often included in public stories. In this setting, Alexander was a symbol for the good Christian, whereas the poison damsel was luxury, lust, and gluttony, which are venomous to the soul (ibid., 27).

Penzer also mentions an interesting twist to the story, wherein a king in India named Mahmud Shah, who lived c. 1500 AD in Gujarat, raised his son on tiny doses of poison to avoid threats of poisoning by his enemies. He was also said to chew different poisonous leaves and spit on whomever he wanted to kill. He was said to have 3000−4000 wives, and whenever he slept with one, she was found dead in the morning (ibid., 31−32).

The American author Nathaniel Hawthorne adapted the poison maiden motif in a story published under the title *Rappacini's Daughter*. In it, according to Penzer, an Italian doctor cruelly uses his newborn daughter for one of his many strange experiments. He begins by having her continually inhale the odor of poisonous plants in his garden, and after some years she becomes immune to the poison. A young man seeks to marry her, and her father devises an antidote to protect him, but she dies from the antidote because of how accustomed she had become to the poison (ibid., 28).

Penzer explores a fascinating array of ideas on the source of the poison damsel motif. Fear of deflowering is one of the most notable, as many cultures had taboos against it, assigning the task to a proxy man who was trained to handle the demonic forces unleashed with the broken hymen. A related motif pointed to by Penzer is that of *vagina dentata*, the primitive psychological fear of vaginal teeth that supposedly drain a man of his vitality (ibid., 44).

Penzer spends the remainder of his article—about a third of it—exploring the possibility that syphilis is behind the motif, a theory that he ultimately dismisses and for good reason: it kills slowly, whereas the venomous virgin always kills relatively instantaneously.

The most recent incarnation of the venomous virgin is the 1991 Bollywood screenplay *Vish Kanyā* (directed by Jag Mundhra), which uses a Hindi version of the original Sanskrit name for the figure. The film, which is available online, but unfortunately without subtitles, is a thriller about a girl (Pooja Bedi) who witnesses her mother's rape and the murder of both parents by a band of Indian mobsters. Her uncle takes her to a local yogi, who gives him poison to feed the girl daily. She grows into a beauty, and is herself raped by an assailant who quickly dies. She escapes to a Kali temple and asks Kali why this has happened, whereupon she remembers her mother's fate and her own mission to seek revenge. She becomes possessed by Kali, lets a cobra bite her hand to no ill effect, and smears the blood on her forehead in place of the usual Hindu auspicious mark. She then sets out on her dangerous mission and successfully seduces and kills each of her parents' attackers in turn.

10.3 CONCLUSION

The venomous virgin motif certainly makes for an excellent story, and connects well with the common cultural tropes of the *femme fatale* and dangerous female sexuality. I should note explicitly that it is an idea spawned by men, for men, and it does not treat women in a respectful manner. It portrays women as simple tools for men to use against each other, even if it spells a life of misery and death for the women themselves.

For Penzer, the poison damsel is a literary motif that was spawned in India over 2000 years ago. He does not believe that it was ever a reality. I, however, see no reason to believe it was not based on some isolated cases in which this really happened. The technique known as mithridatism has become quite well known lately, especially in the context of the life of herpetologist Bill Haast, who injected himself with snake venom for over half of his 101-year life, and credited this to surviving 172 venomous bites. To the end, he was not sure that the venom injections had anything to do with his longevity, but he would not rule it out. Haast also offered transfusions of his blood in place of antivenin to numerous people who had been bitten by snakes for whose poison no antivenin was available. Since antibodies neutralize snake venom, we should rule this out as the food of the venomous virgin. Perhaps plant poison was the basis of her toxic diet. Mithridatism was, of course, well known in ancient India, and medical texts I work with describe conditions under which small amounts of plant poison may even be used medicinally. I leave it to professional toxicologists to decide whether this might translate to a real-life venomous virgin, but the evidence seems strong that it is an original reality that also made for a good story.

REFERENCES

[1] Wujastyk D. The roots of ayurveda: selections from Sanskrit medical writings. New York, NY: Penguin Books; 2003.

[2] Coulson M. *Rākṣasa's Ring*. Clay Sanskrit library. New York, NY: NYU Press; 2005.

[3] Penzer NM. Poison damsels and other essays in folklore and anthropology. Compares tales of the poison damsel from ancient Greece, India, and Europe. London: C.J. Sawyer; 1952.

CHAPTER 11

Mushroom Intoxication in Mesoamerica

Carl de Borhegyi and Suzanne de Borhegyi-Forrest

Bernal Díaz del Castillo, a foot soldier in the army of Conquistador Hernán Cortés, was one of the first Spanish chroniclers to view and describe Tenochtitlan, the Aztec capital and site of modern-day Mexico City. He tells us that the men marveled at the city's size, magnificence, and cleanliness. But while the Spaniards stood in awe of the Aztec's artistic and cultural achievements, they were appalled at their religious ceremonies. These ceremonies included human sacrifice and the consumption of hallucinogenic mushrooms called teonanácatl or "God's flesh." The Spanish friars perceived these entheogenic (god generating) ceremonies to be a horrific, Satan-inspired, and misinterpretation of Christian communion. In the years that followed, the Catholic Church waged a ruthless campaign to stamp out all traces of native religion, and most specifically mushroom worship. During this cultural holocaust they tore down temples, destroyed idols, and burned thousands of colorful hand-painted manuscripts, called codices, dealing with indigenous history and mythology.

The mushroom encountered and described by the Spanish chroniclers was in all likelihood the *Psilocybe cubensis*, the most common of the 40 or so species of Psilocybe mushroom. The hallucinogenic ingredient of this mushroom, as in others of this genus, is psilocybin or psilocin. Somewhat surprisingly, however, this mushroom was not the first and most commonly used hallucinogen. Judging from the many illustrations of sacred mushrooms in ancient Mesoamerican art, some dating back to Olmec times, that distinction may go to the *Amanita muscaria*, or "fly agaric" mushroom of European folklore [1]. The Psilocybe and Amanita mushrooms, along with the equally well known peyote cactus, are only part of a large pharmacopeia of hallucinogens used in Mesoamerica. These include *Datura inoxia* and other species of the genus *Solandra*; a potent species of tobacco called *piciétl* (*Nicotiana rustica*); and the seeds from two morning glories, the white

History of Toxicology and Environmental Health. DOI: http://dx.doi.org/10.1016/B978-0-12-801506-3.00011-X

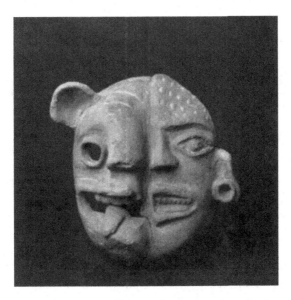

Figure 11.1 "Hidden in plain sight," the ceramic pre-Columbian mask depicts the transformation of a human into a "were-jaguar," a half-human, half-jaguar deity. The were-jaguar appears in the art of the ancient Olmecs as early as 1200 BC The mask symbolizes the soul's journey into the underworld where it will undergo ritual decapitation, jaguar transformation, and spiritual resurrection. Photo courtesy of the International Museum of Ceramics in Faenza, Italy.

flowered *Turbina corymbosa*, and the blue or violet flowered *Ipomoea violacea*, whose active principles are closely allied to synthetic LSD-25. Their psychedelic seeds were considered sacred to the point of divinity [2]. There is mixed evidence for the use of highly poisonous toad toxin. In the mid-seventeenth century the English Dominican friar, Thomas Gage, reported that the Pokoman Maya of Guatemala steeped toads and tobacco in the fermentation of their ritual drink [3]. Whether this mixture was hallucinogenic rather than fatal is, however, a matter of some dispute (Figure 11.1).

In South America the Indians, even more than in Mesoamerica, discovered and experimented with the hallucinogenic properties of plants. They successfully combined unrelated species to activate their psychoactive properties or heighten their effects. Lacking the painstaking ethnography of another chronicler of the Spanish Conquest, Franciscan friar Bernardino de Sahagún, and the medical and botanical compilations of the royal physician Francisco Hernández, anthropologists and mycologists have had to rely heavily on the post-Conquest treatises of Jacinto de la Serna and Ruiz de Alarcón for an understanding of the

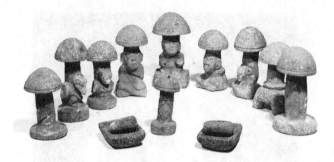

Figure 11.2 Nine Preclassic mushroom stones found in a cache along with nine miniature metates at the highland Maya archaeological site of Kaminaljuyu. The contents of the cache were dated by Stephan de Borhegyi at 1000–500 BC The tall jaguar mushroom stone on the left, also from Kaminaljuyu, was excavated separately. Photo property of author.

continued functions of plant hallucinogens during the early Colonial period (Figure 11.2).

The *Amanita muscaria*, described as poisonous in most scientific literature, is a powerful hallucinogen known from Paleolithic times in northern Europe. The substances muscarine and ibotenic acid are responsible for this mushroom's powerful psychoactive effects. Knowledge of the psychoactive properties of both the Amanita and toad toxin, as well as that of other hallucinogens, was presumably brought to the New World from northeastern Asia by early settlers as a shamanic cult. The magical importance of the Amanita to Mesoamerica is clear from its many portrayals in all Mesoamerican art forms.

In the early 1950s the author's father, archaeologist Stephan F. de Borhegyi, better known by his contemporaries as Borhegyi, wrote the first of a series of articles on the enigmatic small stone sculptures called "mushroom stones" that had turned up in collections and in a few archaeological excavations in the central highlands of Guatemala. Although these artifacts had been known for a number of years, Borhegyi was the first to suspect that they may have been used in an ancient hallucinogenic mushroom cult. After cataloging them by type and provenience, he dated their earliest appearance to approximately 1000 BC According to their archaeological context, mushroom stones were associated from their first appearance with ritual human decapitation, a trophy head cult, warfare and the Mesoamerican ballgame. While mycologists readily accepted this proposition, archaeologists, in

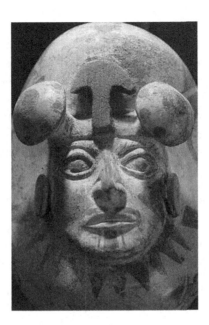

Figure 11.3 A pre-Columbian ceramic Moche portrait vessel from Peru wearing a headdress encoded with two Amanita muscaria mushrooms, together with a mushroom-shaped axe. The Moche culture reigned on the north coast of Peru from 100–600 AD.

general, were dubious. Such reluctance, in the face of much evidence to the contrary, may derive from the deep-seated Western cultural fear of mushroom poisoning combined with a distaste for the excesses of "magic" mushroom experimentation (Figure 11.3).

In an ironic compensation for the terrible loss of indigenous history inflicted by the Catholic Church, Spanish chronicler Bernardino de Sahagún compiled a 12-volume history of New Spain which we know as the Florentine Codex, or *Historia General de las Cosas de Nueva España*. His manuscript is one of the most remarkable ethnographic studies ever assembled, these volumes were the result of decades of research during which Sahagún was aided greatly by his native students. They are located in the Laurentian Library in Florence where they were probably sent by the Inquisition for their content of pagan rituals. When they were discovered in 1883, they became a priceless source of indigenous history, customs, and beliefs.

Sahagún was very likely the first to record the use of hallucinogenic mushrooms in Mesoamerican religion. He writes in Book 9 that merchant groups known as the *pochteca* were devout followers of the god Quetzalcoatl [4]. A passage from the book reads: "...the Indians gathered mushrooms in grassy fields and pastures and used them in religious ceremonies because they believed them to be the flesh of their gods (teonanácatl)." Mushroom intoxication, according to Spanish reports, gave sorcerers the power to seemingly change themselves into animals. The powerful visions and voices the mushrooms produced were believed to be from God. In the Florentine Codex, Sahagún writes:

> *It was said that they did not die {the Indians}, but wakened out of a dream they had lived, this is the reason why the ancients said that when men died, they did not perish, but began to live again, waking almost out of a dream, and that they turned into spirits or gods... and so they said to the dead: "Lord or Lady, wake, for it begins to dawn, now comes the daylight for the yellow-feathered birds begin to sing, and the many colored butterflies go flying,"... and when anyone died, they used to say of him that he was now teotl, meaning to say he had died in order to become a spirit or god.*

Among the many gems of native history preserved by Sahagún is a description of the death of Quetzalcoatl Topiltzin. This great ruler of the city of Tula, the capital of the Toltec empire that preceded the Aztec Empire, was named after their legendary culture hero Quetzalcoatl, also known as the Plumed Serpent. It was the god Quetzalcoatl who they believed had brought all learning and wisdom to the Aztecs and their predecessors.

According to legend, Quetzalcoatl Topiltzin disgraced himself and was banished from his beloved Tula. He traveled southward with a band of his followers, eventually reaching the shores of Yucatan, where he immolated himself and ascended into the heavens as Venus, the Morning Star. The account of Quetzalcoatl's death recorded by Sahagún is quite different and may be closer to historical truth. Sahagún records that, being very ill, Quetzalcoatl was visited by a necromancer who brought him a potion to drink. At first he refused, but after much persuasion he agreed to swallow the potion [5]. Finding the liquid very tasty and pleasant he drank more, only to realize later that he had made a fatal mistake. The contents of the potion have never been identified, but judging from the fact that it caused his death, new evidence would suggest that it was likely the hallucinogenic/toxic *Amanita muscaria* mushroom mixed with honey.

In a guide for missionaries written before 1577, Francisco Hernández de Córdoba, physician to the king of Spain, writes that at the time of the Spanish Conquest, the Aztecs revered three different kinds of narcotic mushrooms [6]. The Spanish Jesuit scholar Jacinto de la Serna (The Manuscript of Serna) later added these words concerning mushroom use in divination:

> These mushrooms were small and yellowish and to collect them the priest and all men appointed as ministers went to the hills and remained almost the whole night in sermonizing and praying [7].

Another renowned Spanish chronicler, Fray Diego Durán, writes in his *Histories of New Spain* (*1537–1588*) that the practice of human sacrifice was the custom that the Spanish considered most shocking. He also writes that mushrooms were used in connection with human sacrifice. Rather than being a punishment, sacrifice was a sacred gift. As he explains, the word for sacrifice, *nextlaoaliztli* in the Nahuatl language of the Aztecs, meant either "payment," or the act of payment (for blessings received). Young children were taught that death by the obsidian knife was a most honorable way to die, as praiseworthy as dying in battle or for a mother and child to die in childbirth. Those who were sacrificed were assured a place in Omeyocan, the paradise of the sun, the afterlife. Quoting Durán:

> The Indians made sacrifices in the mountains, and under shaded trees, in the caves and caverns of the dark and gloomy earth. They burned incense, killed their sons and daughters and sacrificed them and offered them as victims to their gods; they sacrificed children, ate human flesh, killed prisoners and captives of war...It was common to sacrifice men on feast days as it is for us to kill lambs or cattle in the slaughterhouses.... I am not exaggerating; there were days in which two thousand, three thousand or eight thousand men were sacrificed...Their flesh was eaten and a banquet was prepared with it after the hearts had been offered to the devil.... to make the feasts more solemn all ate wild mushrooms which make a man lose his senses...One thing in all this history: no mention is made of their drinking wine of any type, or of drunkenness. Only wild mushrooms are spoken of and they were eaten raw...

Durán called these mushroom ceremonies the "Feast of the Revelations." He also tells us that wild mushrooms were eaten at the ceremony commemorating the accession of the Aztec King Moctezuma in 1502. After Moctezuma took his Divine Seat, captives were brought before him and sacrificed in his honor. He and his attendants then ate a stew made from their flesh.

And all the Lords and grandees of the province. . .all ate of some woodland mushrooms, which they say make you lose your senses, and thus they sallied forth all primed for the dance. . .With this food they went out of their minds and were in worse state than if they had drunk a great quantity of wine. They became so inebriated and witless that many of them took their lives in their hands. With the strength of these mushrooms they saw visions and had revelations about the future, since the devil spoke to them in their madness [8].

In 1951, Borhegyi's research on mushroom stones brought him into contact with amateur ethnomycologist Robert Gordon Wasson, and the two began an extensive correspondence. They both wondered at the pervasiveness of toad effigies on mushroom stones, and the toad's association with the "toadstool" and the ubiquitous appearance of the red and white Amanita muscaria mushroom in northern European folk art. Wasson also called Borhegyi's attention to early Guatemalan dictionary sources describing a mushroom called *xibalbaj ocox*, meaning "underworld mushroom," and *k'aizalab ocox*, meaning "lost judgment mushroom" [3, p. 484].

Soon after their first meeting, Wasson published his account of the modern-day ritual use of hallucinogenic mushrooms among the Mazatec Indians of Oaxaca, Mexico. Wasson's report was followed by similar accounts of hallucinogenic mushroom use among the Zapotec, Chinantec, Mazatec, and Huichol Indians of Mexico. Oddly, although Maya "mushroom stone" sculptures had first suggested the existence of an ancient mushroom cult, evidence for the existence of modern-day mushroom ceremonies in the Maya area appeared to be lacking. Then, in 1972, ethnoarchaeologist Peter Furst reported that Lacandon Maya shamans consumed hallucinogenic mushrooms in the course of their religious ceremonies; and in 1978 ethnomycologist Bernard Lowy reported their intimate association with a creation myth among the Tzutuhil Maya [9].

At about the same time, Michael Coe reported his discovery of numerous toad bones in Olmec burials at San Lorenzo. He suggested that the Olmecs may have used hallucinogenic toad toxin in ritual practices as early as 1200 BC Tatiana Proskouriakoff, graphic artist and illustrator for the Carnegie Institution of Washington archaeological research team, demonstrated that in Mayan glyphs the toad is a symbol of rebirth [3, p. 528]. Furst suggested that the Olmecs may have carried elements of their religion, including a shamanistic supernatural jaguar cult, as well as a mushroom cult, throughout Mesoamerica and even into South America.

In a letter written in 1954 to Wasson, Borhegyi mentions two interesting passages from native chronicles relating to indigenous use of mushrooms in Guatemala: A passage from the *Popol Vuh*, the Quiche Maya Book of Creation reads:

And when they found the young of the birds and the deer, they went at once to place the blood of the deer and of the birds in the mouth of the stones that were Tohil, and Avilix. As soon as the blood had been drunk by the gods, the stones spoke, when the priest and the sacrificers came, when they came to bring their offerings. And they did the same before their symbols, burning pericon (?) and holom-ocox (the head of the mushroom, holom = head, and ocox = mushroom).

He also cites a passage from *The Annals of the Cakchiquels* which records:

At that time, too, they began to worship the devil. Each seven days, each 13 days, they offered him sacrifices, placing before him fresh resin, green branches, and fresh bark of the trees, and burning before him a small cat, image of the night. They took him also the mushrooms, which grow at the foot of the trees, and they drew blood from their ears [10].

Both Wasson and Borhegyi proposed that the mushroom stones were modeled after the *Amanita muscaria* mushroom. Unfortunately, after Borhegyi's premature death in an automobile accident in 1969, further inquiry into the subject on the part of archaeologists came to a virtual halt. It was left to ethnohistorian Peter Furst and a few mycologists, most notably Bernard Lowy and Gaston Guzmán, to continue to make important contributions to the scientific literature.

Gordon Wasson may have provided an important explanation for this lack of interest among archaeologists. He and his Russian wife Valentina had observed that, across the globe, cultures appeared to be divided into those who loved and revered mushrooms, and those who dismissed and feared them. The first group of cultures they labeled "mycophiles," while the latter were "mycophobes." In the New World, it appears that all of the native cultures were, and still are, unquestionably mycophilic. In contrast, the great majority of archaeologists and ethnologists who studied and described them, and who traced their cultural origins to Western Europe, were decidedly mycophobic. This major difference in cultural background may be responsible for what I believe should be seen as a lamentable gap in our understanding of indigenous New World magico-religious origins [11, p. 84–85].

In 1998, I decided to follow up on my father's earlier research on the role of mushrooms in Mesoamerican religion. In this I was aided immensely by Justin Kerr's remarkable compilation and database of roll-out photographs of Mesoamerican art. As a result of this study of Mesoamerican figurines, sculpture, murals, and vase paintings, along with an abundance of evidence from other scholars, I have been able to expand this subject far beyond my father's and Wasson's pioneering efforts.

While I found no mention of images of mushroom stones, pottery mushrooms, or images of actual mushrooms in Kerr's extensive index, I did discover a significant number of images, both realistic and abstract, of both the *Amanita muscaria* and the Psilocybin mushroom. However, it was easy to understand why the imagery had not been noted earlier. On many vases, the images of mushrooms, or images related to mushrooms, were so abstract, and so intricately interwoven with other complex and colorful elements of Mesoamerican mythology and iconography, that they were, quite literally, "hidden in plain sight." This, I believe, was no accident but a deliberate effort to conceal sacred information from the eyes of the uninitiated. As a result, the sacred mushrooms, so cleverly encoded in the religious art of the New World, escaped prior detection. Now after more than a half century of virtual denial by the anthropological community, we have clear visual evidence that two varieties of hallucinogenic mushrooms, the *Amanita muscaria* and the Psilocybin mushroom, as well as the peyote cactus, were worshiped and venerated as gods in ancient Mesoamerica.

Much of the mushroom imagery I discovered was associated with an artistic concept I refer to as underworld jaguar transformation. Under the influence of the hallucinogen, the "bemushroomed" individual is depicted with feline fangs, claws, and spots; attributes of the jaguar as the Underworld Sun God. This esoteric association of mushrooms and jaguar transformation was earlier noted by Furst, together with the fact that a dictionary of the Cakchiquel Maya language compiled *circa* 1699 lists a mushroom called "jaguar ear" [11, p. 80] Many of the mushroom images also involved rituals of self-sacrifice and decapitation in the underworld, alluding to the sun's nightly death and subsequent resurrection by a pair of deities associated with the dualistic nature of the planet Venus as both the Morning star and Evening star. The dualistic aspect of Venus, the brightest "star" in the evening or morning sky, is why this planet was venerated as both a God of Life and God of Death. According to *The Title of the Lords of Totonicapan*, [12] "they [the Quiche] gave thanks to the sun and moon and stars, but particularly to the 'star' that proclaims the day, the day-bringer, the Morning star."

Mushrooms were also so closely associated with death, underworld jaguar transformation, and Venus resurrection in Maya vase paintings, that I conclude that they were likely believed to be the vehicle through which both occurred. They are also so closely associated with ritual decapitation, that their ingestion may have been considered essential to the ritual itself, whether in real life or symbolically in the underworld. It is also important to note that in many cases the mushroom images appeared to be associated with period endings in the Maya calendar.

Gordon Wasson theorized that the origin of ritual decapitation lay in the mushroom ritual itself. In a letter to Borhegyi in 1954 he writes of the Mixe use of the Psilocybin mushroom:

The cap of the mushroom in Mije (or Mixe) is called kobahk, the same word for head. In Kiche and Kakchiquel it is doubtless the same, and kolom ocox is not "mushroom heads," but mushroom caps, or in scientific terminology, the pileus of the mushroom. The Mije in their mushroom cult always sever the stem or stipe (in Mije tek is "leg") from the cap, and the cap alone is eaten. Great insistence is laid on this separation of cap from stem. This is in accordance with the offering of "mushroom head" in the Annals [of the Cakqhiquels] and the Popol Vuh. The writers had in mind the removal of the stems. The top of the cap is yellow and the rest is the color of coffee, with the gills of a color between yellow and coffee. They call this mushroom, pitpa "thread-like," the smallest, perhaps 2 horizontal fingers high, with a cap small for the height, growing everywhere in clean earth, often along the mountain trails with many in a single place. In Mije the cap of the mushroom is called the "head" "kobahk in the dialect of Mazatlan. When the "heads" are consumed, they are not chewed, but swallowed fast one after the other, in pairs [13, 7 June].

In another letter to Borhegyi, Wasson quotes his Mije informant as follows:

The mushrooms may be gathered by anyone at any hour. Often on kneeling to gather one up, the gatherer utters a prayer of thanks for the divine gift. The mushrooms are placed in a jicara, or gourd bowl, and taken to the church. The mushrooms are placed on the high altar, prayers are said, and copal incense is burned. The mushrooms are taken to the house where the session is to be held, perhaps the home of a sick person. The sick person eats the mushrooms, not a curandero: here is the basic difference from the Mazatec practice. If a lost or stolen object is sought, then the suppliant eats the mushroom in the presence of a close member of his family, all others keeping away. The witness is present to give ear to the words of the eater, as he begins to talk under the influence of the inebriating mushrooms. Furthermore, the mushrooms will not render service if he who eats them has said or thought disrespectful things about them, and if he is guilty of this sin, then the mushrooms cause him to see horrible visions of snakes and such like" [13, 19 June].

In 1960, Christian missionary and anthropologist Eunice V. Pike wrote to Borhegyi that Christian missionaries had difficulty in converting the Mazatec Indians because they equated hallucinogenic mushrooms with Jesus Christ. In an earlier letter written in 1953, she elaborated on the subject of Jesus Christ and the mushroom. Note the association of the mushroom with Christ's blood. In Mesoamerican mythology mushrooms were believed to grow where lightning had struck the ground. Water was believed to be god's great gift to mankind; while the sacrificial blood of a human was seen as man's great gift to the gods.

The Mazatecs seldom talk about the mushroom to outsiders, but belief in it is widespread. A twenty-year old boy told me, "I know that outsiders don't use the mushroom, but Jesus gave it to us because we are poor people and can't afford a doctor and expensive medicine...Sometimes they refer to it as "the blood of Christ," because supposedly it grows only where a drop of Christ's blood has fallen. They say that the land in this region is "living" because it will produce the mushroom whereas; the hot dry country where the mushroom will not grow is called "dead." They say that it helps "good people" but if someone who is bad eats it "it kills him or makes him crazy." When they speak of "badness" they mean "ceremonially unclean." (A murderer if he is ceremonially clean can eat the mushroom with no ill effects.) A person is considered safe if he refrains from intercourse five days before and after eating the mushroom. A shoemaker in our part of town went crazy about five years ago. The neighbors say it was because he ate the mushroom and then had intercourse with his wife...When a family decides to make use of the mushroom they tell their friends to bring them any they see, but they ask only those who they can trust to refrain from intercourse at that time, for if the person who gathers the mushroom has had intercourse, it will make the person who eats it crazy [14]."

In conclusion, while indigenous traditions are being lost at a rapid rate everywhere in the world, in Mesoamerica they have thus far proved to be highly resistant to change. Though weakened and almost seamlessly incorporated into Christian beliefs, the use of hallucinogenic substances in native religion has apparently persisted in the more remote areas where they are used in native curing and divination ceremonies. It is precisely the Maya's strong sense of cultural identity that has enabled their communities in Guatemala and Mexico to survive years of discrimination and brutal persecution. In this sense, it can be said that their old Mesoamerican gods are still helping to protect them from evil.

REFERENCES

[1] Borhegyi de CR, De Borhegyi-Forrest S. The genesis of a mushroom/Venus religion in Mesoamerica. In: Rush JA, editor. Entheogens and the development of culture: the anthropology and neurobiology of ecstatic experience. Berkeley, CA: North Atlantic Books; 2013. p. 451–83.

[2] Evans SR, Webster DL, editors. Archaeology of ancient Mexico and Central America: an encyclopedia. 2nd ed. New York, NY: Routledge Publishing; 2010.

[3] Sharer R. [expanded and revised edition of Morley SG, The ancient Maya, 1946] The ancient Maya. 4th ed. Stanford, CA: Stanford University Press; 1983.

[4] Sahagun de Bernardino. Florentine Codex (1540-1585), 12 vols. [Anderson A, Dibble C, Trans. and Ed.]. 1950-1982 Santa Fe, NM: School of American Research

[5] Sahagun de Bernardino. The History of Ancient Mexico [Bandelier F, Trans.] Nashville, TN: Bardwell Printing Co.; 1932. p. 180-1

[6] Serna de la, J. Manual. Para los ministros de indios para el conocimiento de sus idolatrias y extirpacion de ellas. Anals 1900;6:261-80.

[7] Wasson RG, Pau S. The hallucinogenic mushrooms of Mexico and psilocybin, a bibliography. Harvard University Botanical Leaflets 1962;20(2):39.

[8] Wasson RG. The wondrous mushroom: mycolatry. Mesoamerica. New York, NY: McGraw-Hill; 1980. p. 200.

[9] Lowy B. Ethnomycological inferences from mushroom stones. In: Maya codices and Tzutuhil legend. Revista Interamericana 1980;10:94–103.

[10] Borhegyi SF, Wasson RG. Harvard University Botanical Museum, Wasson Archives, 1954.

[11] Furst P. Hallucingens and culture. San Francisco, CA: Chandler and Sharp Publishers; 1976.

[12] Goetz D, Chonay DJ. The title of the lords of Totonicapan. Norman, OK: University of Oklahoma Press; 1974. p. 184.

[13] Wasson RG, Borhegyi SF. Wasson archives. Harvard University Botanical Museum; 1954.

[14] Pike E, letter to Wasson. Wasson Archives Harvard University Botanical Museum; 1953

CHAPTER 12

Entheogens in Ancient Times
Wine and the Rituals of Dionysus

Carl A. P. Ruck

The abuse of psychoactive substances triggered by R. Gordon Wasson's revelations in his *Life* magazine article of May 13, 1957 about drug-induced shamanic rites among the indigenous peoples of the New World, and the subsequent popularization of LSD, which Albert Hofmann had discovered in 1943, made it necessary to create the neologism "entheogen" to discuss the religious role of such substances, divorced from the drug culture of the so-called psychedelic revolution, with its excessive examples of self-indulgence and addiction. An "entheogen" is a mind-altering substance that, as its Greek roots indicate, induces the experience of being *entheos*, in communion with the deity, of sharing an identity with the deity, of having the god dwell within [1]. Entheogens are central to the historical record of humankind's spiritual quest for the meaning of existence, documented in rock paintings as early as the Paleolithic and continuing through all periods in rituals of secret societies and among the ecclesiastical elite of most religions until the present.

Ironically, neither mushrooms nor LSD are, in fact, addictive, nor are many psychoactive agents listed in the Controlled Substances Act (CSA) of 1970 and subsequent amendments classified with a high potential for abuse. The threat that they pose is as a stimulus for political and theological innovation since there is no established context or etiquette for their use, whereas when incorporated into traditional ritual enactments, they can serve the opposite purpose of confirming societal norms or group identities through communal experience of shared metaphysical expectations. The latter was the situation in antiquity.

Although alcoholic beverages were produced and consumed in antiquity, ethanol itself, as a chemical substance, was discovered only in the mid-fourteenth century CE, when the Spanish Franciscan monk

History of Toxicology and Environmental Health. DOI: http://dx.doi.org/10.1016/B978-0-12-801506-3.00012-1

Johannes de Rupescissa succeeded in isolating ethanol from distilled wine. He employed Arabic procedures for processing various metallic substances, such as antimony sulfide, called *koh'l* (kohl) in Arabic and used as an eye cosmetic since antiquity. In the eighth and ninth centuries, Muslim experimenters had used distillation for extracting volatile vapors which they could not capture or contain but which burned upon release as *aqua ardens*, "burning water." Rupescissa named his discovery *aqua vitae*, the "water of life." With the Arabic article *al* it became "alcohol." Rupescissa considered it the *quinta essentia* or "fifth essence," which Aristotle had theorized existed as the elusive substance that permeated and bound together the four elements of fire, air, water, and earth that the fifth-century Empedocles of Acragas had posited as the fundamental materials from which the universe was constructed. Ethanol was immediately greeted as the "spirit molecule" and it quickly spread through philosophical and theological networks as a major advance in chemistry, which later disowned the mystical implications of its origin by separating itself as a science from alchemy.

Early humankind employed a wide variety of toxic substances from botanical and animal sources to alter consciousness in both religious and recreational contexts. Among these were the ferments of sugary liquids, in particular honey, whose inebriating drink was called mead, providing the basic term for "intoxicant" in Greek and yielding the word "mad" in English. Following the discovery of wild grapes with higher sugar contents, fermentation was applied to the crushed juices from the fruit of the vine to produce wine. However, all ferments, that is, mead, beer, and wine, are limited in their content of alcohol by the fact that the natural yeasts that engender fermentation die when the concentration of ethanol makes the liquid too inhospitable for further growth. This occurs at the highest limit of around 14%, which is termed "seven proof" in modern nomenclature, and denotes a drink of moderate intoxicating potential.

Nevertheless, it was customary in antiquity to drink wine diluted with three or four parts water, yielding a drink of around only two proof, which is a quite low alcoholic content. A legendary Thracian wine required 20 parts dilution, and in actuality, a wine that went by that name in the Roman period required 8 parts of water to be drunk safely. Despite the low alcoholic content, wine had a mind-altering potency that could result in complete mental derangement or narcosis after consumption of only four cups over a period of several hours.

Such an effect could not be due to the toxicity of the alcohol. The conclusion of a drinking party often continued out into the streets with public rowdiness and, not infrequently, violent and aggressive behavior [2]. Without dilution, wine might result in permanent brain damage or, as reported on one occasion, even death, which occurred after only 10 cups for a group of young athletes in their physical prime. A Greek drinking cup held about 100 ml. Thus, 10 cups would be a liter.

The virulence of the drink far exceeded its alcoholic content, and was derived from the various fortifying toxins added to it. These included venoms extracted from poisonous animals and insects and from toxic plants, including lethal poisons at dangerously threshold dosages [3]. The use of some drugs, like henbane, was considered age inappropriate and unseemly in an adult but was deemed the sort of thing expectable in a juvenile or pubescent like 'glue-sniffing' today. An ancient comedian said, "Still doing henbane at your age!" Other drugs were reserved for religious contexts, and profane recreational use was sacrilegious and punishable by death. Among the toxins added to the wine, identifiable agents include serpent and salamander venoms, hemlock, jimsonweed, aconite, cannabis, wormwood, ergot, and probably dimethyltryptamine (DMT) from acacia and similar plants, as well as psychoactive resins and incenses. Other toxins are masked under names that probably refer to special compounded mixtures. Just recently, in 2013, a storeroom of still-extant wine dating from the mid-second millennium BCE that was unearthed in Canaan, excavation site of Tel Kabri, near kibbutz Kabri, Israel, confirms the presence of psychoactive additives, which previously was documented only in literary texts [4].

Since opium was among the additives, addiction was inevitable, and persons were satirized for drunkenness and overindulgence. The low alcoholic content of diluted wine probably precluded the possibility of actual alcoholism in most cases, and the perceived dependency was due to the toxic additives. This is probably true even of those individuals who were said to have indulged in drinking their wine unmixed, in the Thracian fashion, to the point of permanent derangement or madness. Insanity is the outcome of only the most severe alcoholic addiction. Several prominent figures, especially philosophers, chose to end their lives by drinking. A cup of purely alcoholic wine is hardly appropriate as a means for intentional suicide. However, wine was also the customary way for administering medicinal preparations.

The vessels for the drink involved in certain religious initiations each had a characteristic design, differing from the wine cups of the symposium. They were appropriately larger to hold the complete dosage required for the experience, and the potion was probably not drunk over an extended period of conviviality.

Wine was associated with a particular deity and his analogues in other cultures. By the Classical period, which was the fifth century BCE in Athens, this was the god Dionysus, also known as Bacchus, and there was a complex etiquette or social norm surrounding his worship and the consumption of his drink. The civilized product resulting from the controlled, recognizably fungal growth of the fermenting yeasts was contrasted with the wild naturally occurring toxins, among which mushrooms, containing psychoactive psilocybin and muscimol, and ergot of grain containing lysergic acid amine, played a fundamental role as similarly fungal. The wine drink with its toxic additives was seen as mediating between the dichotomy of natural or wild toxins and their evolution or taming through the art of viticulture. A similar civilizing fungal growth was recognized in the leavening yeasts of bread, linking Dionysus and his analogues with the goddesses of the grain, Demeter and her daughter Persephone, and their analogues, as well as with the netherworld realm of Hades and the afterlife, either chthonic in the blessed fields of Elysium or celestial in the empyrean beyond the solar disk [5]. The entheogen derived from ergot figured in the visionary potion of the Eleusinian Mystery, which was a religious initiation that began in the mid-second millennium and lasted until the Christians persecuted its practitioners and destroyed the sanctuary in the fourth century. It was an experience that afforded meaning to human existence in the context of spiritual dimensions and was something that most of the great thinkers, writers, artists, and politicians of the Greco-Roman world had undergone.

The etiquette of drinking involved different scenarios for men and women and different locales, either within the city or without. For the men, the ritual was the *symposium*, a "communal drinking," or what one might call a cocktail party today. The best-documented exemplar, apart from the numerous depictions on the mixing vessels and cups for the event, is Plato's *Symposium* dialogue. The men gathered at the house of the host and drank a succession of toasts, while engaged in discussion of a proposed topic. The host determined the admixtures, the rate of dilution, and the frequency and number of rounds. Throughout their increasing inebriation, the guests were challenged to maintain sobriety, although even in Plato's symposium, where the men had decided to drink abstemiously since they were still drunk from the previous day, all the guests except Socrates, the comedian Aristophanes, and the tragedian Agathon end up unconscious until dawn.

The characteristic cup for the symposium was the *kylix*, and its design as a broad saucer supported by a narrow stem challenged the drinkers to maintain decorous sobriety since it would be unstable in drunken hands. Dionysus himself never drank from such a vessel, but rather from a double-handled mug called a *kantharos*, which held about a half liter. In addition to its depiction on vase paintings, several fine exemplars survive, probably intended as dedicatory offerings to the deity.

Customarily, a hired female, who sang, danced erotically, and played music, provided entertainment, which often included engaging in sexual activity with the guests. The men, moreover, were usually seated with their male lovers and engaged with each other, as well as with the female professional companion.

The symposium celebrated Dionysus in his avatar as the wine. The women's celebration honored the manifestations of the deity that predated viticulture. For them, he was Bacchus and they became bacchantes. Although customarily secluded in the women's quarters of their homes and subjected to the dominance of their husbands, they left their houses and assembled outside the city in a locale symbolic of the wilderness, typically a mountainside. This was not a place for viticulture, especially in the winter season of the ritual, but instead was where wild herbs abounded, particularly mushrooms. These women were also called madwomen or maenads because of the extreme state of ecstasy they experienced. This involved delusional fantasies of sexual abandon to the amorous onslaught of hybrid creatures imagined as ithyphallic goat-men or satyrs, who represented the spirits of the wilderness and its herbal toxins. Often the god himself was thought to materialize among them as their divine lover, cross-dressing as a female. This hallucinatory reality is well documented in both literary sources and in numerous vase paintings (Figure 12.1). The women also beat tambours, played instruments, and danced, creating a terrifying din of movement and sound. On one occasion documented in a historical record, they descended from the mountain in such a state of

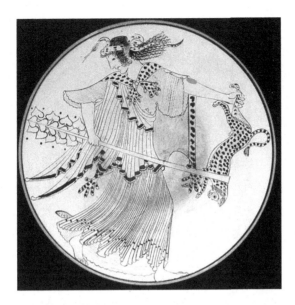

Figure 12.1 Maenad, with thyrsus, stuffed with ivy leaves, holding a leopard and wearing a leopard skin, with snake bound in her hair. Attic white-ground kylix *490-480 BCE, from Vulci, an Etruscan site north of Rome. Collection of the Staatliche Antikensammlungen, Munich, Germany.*

derangement that they fell unconscious in the center of a village and had to be protected through the night from sexual molestation by a garrison of soldiers.

The bacchantes were never depicted drinking wine, since that was not the source of their intoxication. The emblem of their mountain celebration indicates the nature of their ritual activity. This is the *thyrsus*, the long hollow reed of the giant fennel, into which leaves of ivy have been stuffed and are seen protruding from its top (Figure 12.2). It was customary for herb gatherers to use such an implement as the container for the wild plants that they gathered. The maenads were enacting a mimesis of herb gathering, and the object of their quest was symbolized as the wild ivy. It was a plant seen as the primordial vine from which the grapevine was hybridized. Its leaves and berries induced mental derangement in their natural state, without the civilizing intervention of viticulture to tend and prune the vine as necessary to induce it to fruit with the grapes from which the new intoxicant could be manufactured through the process of fermentation. The thyrsus was also called a *narthex*, which is the name of the giant fennel reed, but it also has a transparently obvious etymology as the "container" (*thex*) for the "narcotic" or drug/entheogen.

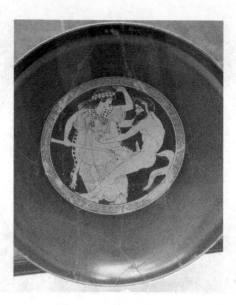

Figure 12.2 Maenad with thyrsus, dueling with ithyphallic satyr, Attic red-figure kylix, *480 BCE Collection of the Staatliche Antikensammlungen, Munich, Germany.*

The prototypic primordial plant symbolized by the leaves of ivy and similar wild vines like bryony (cucumber) and smilax (bindweed) was the uncultivable psychoactive mushroom. Thus, in ordinary culinary nomenclature, the stipe or stem of a mushroom was called its thyrsus. This is a terminology that appears to have been in use for at least a millennium. The fungal cap spreading above the thyrsus represents the toxic herbs gathered into its container. In the case of the *Amanita* mushrooms that yield the visionary muscimol, the psychoactive toxin is primarily confined to the rind of its cap. Both bryony and smilax contain tropane alkaloids that yield LSA (lysergic acid amide, a precursor to LSD).

It is well documented as a folkloric motif that magical plants require special procedures to address or appease their indwelling spirits as rituals for their gathering. The scenario for the bacchante revel indicates the delusional fantasies enacted by the women. They marshaled themselves into generic groupings according to age, as pubescent, maternal, or postmenopausal, and sexually seduced the plant, which in the case of the mushroom was a common metaphor for the penis. The dominant theme is the hunt for the animate manifestation of the plant, typically an animal like the bunny with prolific sexual connotations, the bull with its aggressive masculinity, or the wolf for the shamanic motif of the werewolf transmogrification. They are never depicted, however, with any implements like a net or a trap for the hunt, and they never received instruction for the activity, which was not an ordinary female pursuit. The spirit of the plants materialized and sexually engaged with them. As the primitive antecedent to the grapevine, the plant's proper role was to yield to its civilized successor. The original plant was portrayed as a sacrificial victim, probably in earlier times an actual human offering, whose raw flesh they tasted. The manner of the slaughter was termed a rending apart (or *sparagmos*) with bare hands, but this was hardly likely to be anything more than a metaphor in the case of so powerful and dangerous a beast as a bull. Instead, he bull must be interpreted, like all the other supposed victims, as a fantasized zoomorphic persona of the gathered plant. Thus, the plant was also mothered by the bacchantes as their baby, which they tore to pieces, although there is no evidence that they ever took their own children to the mountain revel. They did, however implausibly, nurse wild animals as their babies. Obviously, the women could not have hunted and caught these animals except as zoomorphic animating personae of the magical plants.

The thyrsus in the lore of the mythological tradition was also the container in which the titan Prometheus concealed the fire that he stole from the celestial gods and entrusted to mankind as the drug that set humans upon their path to consciousness, making them like unto gods. This was the primordial entheogen. Not surprisingly, the bacchantes were also said to handle fire in their hands without being burnt, since the fire is also a metaphor.

The actual source of the toxins that induced their extreme delusional state and ecstasy may have been the serpents that they are frequently depicted handling. One historical account describes stroking the cheeks of the serpents,[1] which would indicate the method for milking the venom, which would then probably be applied as a dermal agent in sexual mimesis since ingestion in most cases would destroy the toxins.

By the Roman period, the bacchantes' revel had broadened to include men. A notorious event in the year 186 BCE is recorded both in

---

[1]On milking snake venoms: Demosthenes, *De corona*, 18.260. On vaginal application of serpent venoms: Juvenal, *Satires*, 6.314–319. On anal application of serpent venoms: Prudentius, *Peristephanon*, 13.21 et seq.

the historical record and in the surviving inscription that preserves the decree of the senate known as the *senatus consultum de Bacchanalibus*, which attempts to limit the rites which had spread from the Greek colonies in the south of the Italian peninsula and had reached as far as the city of Rome. The allegations indicate that women and their knowledge of drugs were originally the dominant source, but that the rites, in addition to actual sexual profligacy, involved the sodomizing of young men and even their sacrificial murder.

In Greece during the Classical age, the symposium of the men was countered by the bacchanalia of the girls and women. The god of the wine was the ultimate mediator between realms, bringing the wild into balance with civilization. Thus a further ritual of etiquette for the drinking of his intoxicant was celebrated as the February festival of the *Anthesteria*. This enacted the opening of the fermented vats of the new wine. Here the drinking was from individual pitchers containing about 700 ml and apparently intended as the probable daylong dosage. As the god returned from his apparent sojourn in the subterranean world, he brought with him all the ghosts of the departed to join in a communal feast with their still-living relatives. This was a reunion that brought the whole family together, not only the living and the dead but also husbands with their wives, their children and their nubile daughters exposed to public view, and even the babies. The latter were given their first taste of wine at the tender age of three or four, and they were indoctrinated into the metaphysical symbolism of the drink. The children are depicted on the characteristic toy-sized drinking pitchers for the festival playing in the vicinity of the gravestones or impersonating their elders in performing some of the most sacred rituals in honor of the god [6].

The festival lasted three days and the drinking induced a state of mind that was parodied on the comic stage as delusional. Despite the drunkenness, the experience was accorded a positive potential. It included humorous attempts to demonstrate sobriety by standing upon a greased wineskin, and in the mythological lore, it coincided with the cure of Orestes from the pursuit of the demons who maddened him, pursuing him for the murder of his mother. It set the precedent for the superior claim of the father over the mother as the parent of the child.

The supreme gift of the deity of intoxication was his patronage of the theater. In the sixth century, under the tyrant Pisistratus, what had begun as a mushroom cult celebrated in the rural mountain villages was imported into the city of Athens. It eventually developed into the theatrical festivals of comedy and tragedy, which made the city into the cultural icon that has assured its role as the fountainhead of the Classical tradition. The hallucinatory realities of the stage enactments were a prime instrument in indoctrinating the populace into the lore of their mythological heritage. Throughout the several days of daylong performances, the audience drank a specially doctored wine, facilitating the pretense of thespian impersonation and blurring the boundaries of imagined and real.

Of the two types of performances, tragedies enacted the motif of the necessary demise of the primitive as fundament for the civilized, essentially the theme of the bacchantes' revel. The comedies, on the other hand, took a different view. They held a finger up to the world and imagined a paradise where baser instincts had their way. Reality could be molded with the fickleness of the phallus and the inexhaustible metaphors it traditionally inspires. Mediating between these two extremes was still another genre of the theater, called the satyr play after the costuming of its dancers. Here the theme was the stories of tragedy, but they were treated as parody with comic intent.

Within the context of the entire cycle of Dionysian events, the intoxication served to reinforce societal norms and cultural identity, but the aggressive rowdiness of drunken ithyphallic symposiasts also roused suspicion of seditious intent aimed at the established political authority.

REFERENCES

[1] Ruck C, Bigwood J, Staples D, Ott J, Wasson R. Entheogens. J Psychedelic Drugs 1979;11 (1−2):145−6.

[2] Rinella M. Pharmakon: Plato, drug culture, and identity in ancient Athens. Lanham, MD: Lexington Books; 2010.

[3] Hillman D. The chemical muse: drug use and the roots of western civilization. New York, NY: St. Martin's Press; 2008.

[4] Associated Press Article, Brandeis University. Archaeologists discover largest, oldest wine cellar in Near East. Science Daily, November 22, 2013.

[5] Ruck C. Sacred mushrooms of the goddess: secrets of Eleusis. Berkeley, CA: Ronin Publishing; 2006.

[6] Wasson R, Hofmann A, Ruck C. The road to Eleusis: unveiling the secret of the mysteries. New York, NY: Harcourt Brace Jovanovich, Inc.; 1978.

CHAPTER 13

Entheogens (Psychedelic Drugs) and the Ancient Mystery Religions

Mark A. Hoffman

13.1 PHARMACOLOGICAL ROOTS OF RELIGION

The Mystery Religions of the ancient world frequently, if not always, employed the use of psychoactive drugs or "entheogens" to induce profound altered states of consciousness. Such experiences were indispensible to the initiation of members, their rituals relating to spiritual development, and ultimately the attainment of the "peak" experience(s) that represented the apotheosis and fulfillment of their theological and spiritual aspirations.

Thus, more than any other principle, the entheogenic—i.e., pharmacological—induction of nonordinary states defines the theology and practice of the ancient Mystery Religions.

A significant body of scholarly data has been applied to attempts to identify specific entheogens used throughout the ages in the Classical Mystery Religions as well as among the early developmental stages of the historical religions (i.e., those thought to be based in some part, at least, upon historical events). Thus, the mythology, art history, and canonical, apocryphal, and historical literary traditions of religions including Judaism, Christianity, Islam, Buddhism, and Hinduism have been shown to contain evidence for entheogenic practices.

Drawing upon ancient sources, religious-comparative evidence, and modern scientific data, it has been possible to identify, with varying degrees of certainty, a range of substances that are likely to have been ritually used to induce altered states of consciousness. The following is a necessarily cursory survey of some of the best documented and historically significant of these religions and their probable use of specific entheogens in a toxicological context, extrapolating likely scenarios relating to the symptomatology of practical entheogenic initiation and

History of Toxicology and Environmental Health. DOI: http://dx.doi.org/10.1016/B978-0-12-801506-3.00013-3

how such effects were interpreted by the initiates and those facilitating the experience.

The original dominance of ancient entheogenic sacramentalism has survived as deeply entrenched and culturally celebrated mythopoetic remnants regarding magical foods and beverages. Christianity has the Eucharist, referencing the blood and body of Christ; Judeo-Christianity, the Forbidden Fruit of the Tree of Knowledge, and manna of heaven; while Buddhism and Sikhism preserve a tradition of imbibing *amrita* (from Sanskrit "immortality") and Taoism has maintained an alchemical tradition regarding an elixir (or mushroom, or fruit) of immortality. The Vedic roots of Hinduism (and Buddhism) and the Iranian/Persian religions, including Islam and Sufism, emerged largely from a shared Indo-European sacramental culture steeped in the sacraments, *soma* and *haoma* (from Proto-Indo-European "pressed" or "pounded") respectively, which contributed to the survival of entheogenic themes in their practices and mythologies.

Prior to the historical religions, and within the cultural and mythopoetic contexts from which they derived, the mythologies of the mystery traditions abound with evidence of magical herbs capable of inducing "immortality" and frequently sought by gods and heroes.

13.2 HERMENEUTICS AND A DEFINITION OF TERMS

"The Mystery Religions" is a somewhat inadequate general phrase that usually denotes the dominant yet diverse religious practices of the ancient Greek and Roman periods. Similar confusion results from the use of the phrase "Classical civilizations," which may either refer specifically to the ancient Greco-Roman world, or to any of the highly developed cultures of the ancient world. For the purposes of this chapter, we extend the meaning to include any of the popular ancient cults that were characterized by ritual secrecy and initiation.

As a side note, it is important to clarify that although this chapter may be a bit beyond the scope of mainstream Western toxicology, it is still quite relevant. Psychoactive substances capable of inducing rarified states of consciousness, which some today might refer to as "intoxication," have a role to play in our historical understanding of toxic agents.

We use the word *entheogen*, first coined in 1976 [1], to describe substances that would be inadequately termed "psychoactive" or "hallucinogenic." While "psychoactive" encompasses all substances and means of "affecting the mind," entheogens are specifically substances that have been used to induce experiences that are considered "spiritual" by those who imbibe them. They previously were called "hallucinogens" in the scientific literature, but many specialists have chosen to abandon this woefully inadequate term in favor of "psychedelic" and/or "entheogenic" in order to avoid the explicit connotation of "illusory" or "false or deluded perceptions" carried by "hallucinogen."

"Entheogen" overcame the inability of other misnomers and neologisms to properly convey "transcendent and beatific states of communion with deity," and more accurately describe these states within the cultural contexts in which they were and are used. An entheogen has also been defined as "any substance that, when ingested, catalyzes or generates an altered state of consciousness deemed to have spiritual significance." The entheogenic epiphany often involves the experience of the dissolution of distinctions or boundaries between the individual and the mystical or supernatural dimensions of the universe, and a sense of direct communion with pure and primal consciousness or divinity [2]. Thus, in addition to its theological implications, "entheogen" also carries a distinctly gnostic or deist connotation that implies a direct, unmediated experience of deity, and shares many attributes in common with shamanic practices and belief systems. A general effect of entheogens is high-voltage, slow-wave, synchronous brain activity that is said to increase the connectivity between the emotional and behavioral brain centers, and between lower-brain areas and the frontal cortex, which occurs primarily via serotonin, dopamine, and mesolimbic disinhibition [3]. These effects on the brain provide an observable basis for the therapeutic use of entheogens and the universality of ecstatic shamanic phenomenology. Therapeutic effects include the activation of emotional processes of the limbic system and paleomammalian brain relating to attachment, emotive responses, and social cohesion [4].

Another important aspect of entheogen-inspired experience, and one especially relevant to ancient Mystery Religions, is that of infusing the initiates' mythological framework with a tangibly new, more immediate, and more profound meaning. One author describes this process as the way in which the "supernatural becomes natural" [5], and Sigmund Freud described the psychiatric use of psychedelics as a way to "make conscious the unconscious" [6, p. 314]. Perhaps the eminent chemist Alexander Shulgin puts it most simply when he wrote that these (psychedelic) compounds, "have given me ... a personal understanding of just who I am and why I am" [7].

Those who ingest entheogenic substances often describe the effects in terms of experiencing as if through a "spectator ego," "where he or she experiences a bond with nature and society, a sense of overwhelming revelation and truth, and a vivid awareness of his or her surroundings" [8].

As scholars of mysticism and comparative religious studies have noted for some decades, the descriptions of mystical union and spiritual ecstasy are often indistinguishable from those induced by means of entheogens. While this fact alone is highly suggestive of a cross-cultural entheogenic component, in many (or even most) cases, an entheogen is directly or indirectly implicated within the history of a spiritual tradition itself. Though the identity of specific entheogens utilized in a given rite may be formulaically veiled, the prominence of place reserved for such sacraments within a given religious tradition follows from the fact that entheogenic experiences often have a profound and life-changing impact upon the initiate, affecting their beliefs and behaviors, and are frequently considered one of the peak experiences of initiates' lives [9].

In the case of the Eleusinian Mysteries of ancient Greece, a sacred potion was given to the initiates, and among the Vedic Indo-European peoples, the *soma* and *haoma* sacraments were consumed in order to gain spiritual insight, inspiration, and poetic prowess. In these cases, the identity of the specific sacrament was kept in highest secrecy, much like the alchemical Philosopher's Stone, as a cult secret to be closely guarded in order to avoid the profanation of their most sacred principles, and to not offend the divine spirit residing within the sacrament.

While a scientific, nonspeculative, toxicological assessment of the mystery sacraments is impossible given the dearth of knowledge regarding the specific compounds and combinations used in a given mystery rite, the use of certain sacramental plants and fungi is well documented in antiquity, and reasonable hypotheses can be extrapolated by means of multidisciplinary inquiries that employ data from fields as wide ranging as botany, chemistry, archaeology, ethnology, comparative religious studies, mythology, and art history.

In addition to perplexing pharmacological questions, we are confronted with problems related to the academic study of hermetic subjects, in this case Mystery Religions that employed "holy" or "sacred" sacraments. Not only are the specific and unique rites veiled in mystery due to a characteristic and pervasive secrecy, but the mystical states of consciousness with which we are concerned can be highly variable and subjective, especially once removed from their "set and setting" within the cultic context.

13.3 TOXICOLOGY

In the context of the ancient Mystery Religions, scholarly consensus holds that the "abuse" and mundane "recreational" use of entheogens in antiquity was, with few exceptions, impracticable, a fact largely due to the cultural context in which they were set, and the often-extreme secrecy regarding their plant sources and the specifics having to do with their preparation. Certainly, this perspective is valid in the sense that the cultic "set and setting," which included ritual preparations and proscriptions, was antithetical to the development of a profane "drug culture," but this is not to say the use of entheogens was limited to the cultic setting. In fact, the evidence for the widespread use of all manner of intoxicants in the ancient world [10] contributes to a better understanding of the likely roles they played in the Mysteries. Another important consideration is that, generally speaking, the primary entheogenic compounds simply aren't addictive, and therefore they are not substances of "abuse."

While some of the entheogens discussed herein are known to cause undesirable physiological side effects, the psychospiritual and therapeutic benefits attributed to these experiences far outweigh the relatively benign and fleeting "toxicity" that may, at times, accompany them. This was as true among ancient initiates as it is today among contemporary practitioners. Thus, for instance, transient nausea, cramps, vomiting, or diarrhea is considered a relatively minor inconvenience when compared to the profundity of experiencing what was considered a direct contact with one's deity or deities in an ecstatic communion—an experience that is thought by many to sacralize, heal, inform, and reintegrate the sacred into the profane, and the individual with group psychospiritual dynamics.

Difficult psychological experiences, usually also transitory but sometimes becoming a major or even dominant side effect of a given 'bad trip," can occur. These are relatively rare and are much more likely to take place in individuals with a history of mental instability, or by individuals with highly ordered, inflexible, or rigid personalities [6, p. 315], an exaggerated or narcissistic ego, and moderate to severe psychological disorders.

Problems also occur more often when entheogens are taken outside of a ritual context, and without the supervision and support of an experienced facilitator. In such cases, self-preparation of the drug can result in an inferior preparation, and self-administration can result in overdose and severe psychological and physiological symptoms.

One side effect of entheogenic "toxicity" commonly mentioned is "panic attacks," for which benzodiazepines or other sedative drugs are often indicated in current medical protocol; it is often also suggested that the medical professional provide a "supportive environment." Such symptoms, usually transitory, can also include fear, depression/despair, anxiety, and tension. Along with the physiological discomforts which might occur, these comprise most of what is known as the "ordeal" aspect of initiations, which in the context of the whole experience would have been considered a valuable and therapeutic component of initiation that introduces humility and additional meaning, perspective, and emotional impact to the experience. Thus, mild to moderate symptomatic difficulties would not necessarily have been considered antithetical, nor would they likely have been treated. Special medical attention would have been relatively uncommon or even rare, and been reserved for the treatment of acute symptomatology, such as extreme pain, vomiting, diarrhea/dehydration, anaphylaxis, or other serious allergic reaction, serotonin syndrome, or the onset of a psychotic adverse reaction (otherwise known as a "freakout") where the initiate might hurt themselves or others and disrupt the ritual.

In the ancient context, as today, the facilitators of entheogenic initiations would have been intimately aware of the wide range of potential effects of these drugs and would have developed both psychological and pharmacological treatments to address especially problematic symptomatology. While the psychological "treatment" would have been consistent with the theological and ritual expectations of the ongoing initiation, physical treatment might have included proactive herbal preparations, massage, movement, emetics, counseling, supervision, and restraint and other methods.

The complexity and vagaries regarding the physiological and neurophysiological actions of specific and combined phytochemicals generally indicates an advanced practical knowledge of pharmacology, dosage, and toxicology. Though much can be learned about the theological characteristics of a religion's entheogenic-sacramental complex, as much can be gleaned by studying the surviving, and surprisingly widespread, shamanic uses of these and similar substances.

13.4 SOURCES, CHEMISTRY, AND EFFECTS

Although entheogenic substances are found in a wide variety of flora, fauna, and fungi, their effects derive from similar chemical compounds known as *indoleamines* that variously affect the brain's neurotransmitter systems. The major classes of indoleamines, tryptamines (e.g., DMT, psilocin, and psilocybin), and phenylethylamines (e.g., mescaline, MDA) exert similar influences on serotonergic neurons.

Thus entheogens can be classified and grouped by chemical structure, as well as the compounds from which they are derived. Chemically related substances tend to exhibit similar effects. Other entheogenic compounds are sometimes termed "pseudohallucinogens" in the medical literature because they are said to produce psychotic and delirious effects without the classic visual disturbances of true hallucinogens. This classification is of limited use for our purposes, however, as various entheogens were/are combined, and the entheogenic nature of an experience is determined within a subjective cultural context. The experience also differs qualitatively even within the same culture, by means of multiple initiatory rituals associated with different classes of entheogens. Thus, for instance, the Huichol Indians of Mexico employ various entheogens at various times for various purposes [11].

Below is a very cursory survey of some specific compounds and their natural sources that were thought to have been used as primary ingredients or admixtures in various mystery sacraments. Other important psychoactive and potentiating plants such as opium and cannabis are also strongly implicated, but will be omitted from the discussion for the sake of brevity.

13.4.1 Amanita Muscaria: "Poison" Apple of the Inner Eye

The psychoactive Amanita mushrooms, specifically *A. muscaria* and *A. pantherina*, have a well-attested entheogenic use among Siberian, European, and Pan-American shamanic peoples and are specifically implicated in the Mysteries of ancient Greece (especially the Mysteries of Dionysus), Rome (Mithraic Mysteries) [12], and as the original Vedic plant-god *soma* [13], and Avestan *haoma* among the gnostic Manicheans and early and mystically inclined Christians of later periods [14].

The unique and striking morphology of these "fairytale" mushrooms can often be an important clue to deciphering veiled, yet sometimes obvious, literary or art-historical references to the use of these important entheogens within certain mystery traditions. The decarboxylation of the often "toxic" muscarine levels of these amanitas, which is largely achieved by drying the fruiting bodies, results in the production of muscimole, the desired nontoxic entheogenic compound. The chemical properties of these mushrooms thus serve as a metaphor for the Mysteries more generally, i.e., when the secret of their preparation is known and applied, the "mystery" contained within them is revealed.

13.4.2 Ergot Alkaloids: A Grail Quest

A preparation of ergot alkaloids is strongly implicated as the key ingredient in the *kykeon* potion of the Greater Eleusinian Mystery, but the safe and practical process for its preparation in ancient times is yet to be rediscovered [15]. Due to the dangerous toxicological effects of some ergot alkaloids and the uncertainties associated with applying chemical techniques available in antiquity, very few human bioassays of possible ancient "recipes" have occurred, and the sound theoretical research remains speculative.

13.4.3 Psilocybin and Psilocin (Mushrooms) and DMT, 5Meo DMT: Spirit Molecules

These closely related entheogenic compounds should be mentioned in a discussion of the Mystery Religions. While evidence for their use in this context has not been fully explored, it is extremely unlikely that the chemical properties of psychoactive mushrooms and the natural sources of DMT would have been overlooked by ancient herbalists and alchemists.

13.4.4 Tropane Alkaloids

While it is highly debatable whether, and to what extent, the tropane-containing plants were used as primary ingredients in mystery sacraments *per se*, they deserve a special mention in terms of toxicity as pharmacologically hazardous compounds. Used as a supplement by contemporary preparers of ayahuasca to their DMT/betacarboline brew, the dosage tropane additives must be carefully controlled in order to avoid acute and long-term deleterious effects. Atropine, scopolamine, and hydrocine, and perhaps other tropane alkaloids, are said to enhance and intensify the affects of compounds such as opium, cannabis, and other entheogenic compounds. Tropane alkaloids were and are used as primary ingredients for shamanic initiations among a number of the shamanic peoples of the Americas and were key ingredients in the medieval witches' "flying ointments."

ADDITIONAL READINGS

Barile F. Clinical toxicology, principles and mechanisms. 2nd ed. Boca Raton, FL: CRC Press; 2010.

Dobkin MD. Hallucinogens: cross-cultural perspectives. Albuquerque, NM: University of New Mexico Press; 1984.

Fantegrossi W, Mernane K, Reissig C. The behavioral pharmacology of hallucinogens. Behav Pharmacol 2008;75:17–33.

Griffiths RR, Richards WA, McCann U, Jesse R. Psilocybin can occasion mystical-type experiences having substantial, sustained personal meaning and spiritual significance. Psychopharmacology 2006;187(3):268–83.

Harner MJ, editor. Hallucinogens and shamanism. New York, NY: Oxford University Press; 1973.

McKenna T. Food of the Gods: the search for the original tree of knowledge. New York, NY: Bantam Books; 1992.

Nichols D. Hallucinogens. Pharmacol Ther 2004;101:131–81.

Nichols D, Chemel B. The neuropharmacology of religious experience. In: McNamara P, editor. Where God and science meet: how brain and evolutionary studies alter our understanding of religion. Westport, CT: Praeger; 2006.

Ott J. Pharmacotheon: entheogenic drugs, their plant sources and history. 1993.

Ruck C, Staples B, Celdran J, Hoffman M. The hidden world: survival of pagan shamanic themes in European fairytales. Durham, NC: Carolina Academic Press; 2007.

Ruck CAP, Staples BD, Heinrich C. The apples of Apollo: pagan and Christian mysteries of the Eucharist. Durham, NC: Carolina Academic Press; 2001.

Schultes R, Hofmann A. Plants of the Gods. New York, NY: McGraw-Hill; 1979.

Wasson G. The wondrous mushroom: mycolatry in Mesoamerica. New York, NY: McGraw-Hill; 1980.

Wasson RG, Kramrisch S, Ott J, Ruck CAP. Persephone's quest: entheogens and the origins of religion. New Haven, CT: Yale University Press; 1986.

REFERENCES

[1] Ruck CAP, Bigwood J, Staples D, Ott J, Wasson G. Entheogens. J Psychedelic Drugs 1976;11(1-2):145−6.

[2] Hoffman M, Ruck CAP. Entheogens (psychedelic drugs) and shamanism. In: Walter MN, Fridman JN, editors. Shamanism: an encyclopedia of world beliefs, practices and culture, vol. I. Santa Barbara, CA: ABC-CLIO; 2004. p. 111−7.

[3] Winkelman M., Hoffman M. Hallucinogens and Entheogens. In Segal R., von Stuckrad K., editors: Vocabulary of religion. Amsterdam: Brill. [forthcoming].

[4] Winkelman M. Psychointegrators: multidisciplinary perspectives on the therapeutic effects of hallucinogens. Complement Health Pract Rev 2001;6(3):219−37.

[5] Winkelman M, Baker J. *Supernatural as natural: a biocultural approach to religion.* Pearson North America, Upper Saddle River, New Jersey; 2008.

[6] Hanson GR, Venturelli PJ, Fleckenstein AE. Drugs and society. 10th ed. Sudbury, MA: Jones and Bartlett; 2009 [cites Snyder 1974. P. 44].

[7] Shulgin A, Perry W. Simple plant isoquinolines. Berkeley, CA: Transform Press; 2002 Pg. iv.

[8] <http://informahealthcare.com/doi/abs/10.3109/9781420092264.016>.

[9] Fadiman J. Psychedelic explorer's guide: safe, therapeutic and sacred journeys. Rochester, VT: Park Street Press; 2001.

[10] Hillman DCA. The chemical muse: drug use and the roots of western civilization. New York, NY: Thomas Dunne Books, St. Martin's Press; 2008.

[11] Hoffman M. Huichol wolf shamanism and *A. muscaria*. In: Hoffman M, editor. Entheos: Journal of Psychedelic Spirituality, vol. 1. 2002. p. 2.

[12] Ruck CAP, Hoffman M, Celdran JG. Mushrooms, myth and Mithras: the drug cult that civilized Europe. San Francisco, CA: City Lights; 2011.

[13] Wasson G. Soma: divine mushroom of immortality. New York, NY: Harcourt, Brace & Jovanovich; 1968.

[14] Hoffman M, Ruck CAP, Staples DB. Conjuring Eden: art and the entheogenic vision of paradise. In: Hoffman M, editor. Entheos: Journal of Psychedelic Spirituality, vol. 1. 2000. p. 1.

[15] Wasson G, Ruck CAP, Hofmann A. The road to Eleusis: unveiling the secret of the mysteries. New York, NY: Harcourt, Brace & Jovanovich; 1978.

Printed in the United States
By Bookmasters